Debrief

True Stories of Advocating for Patients, Building Resilience, and Finding Your Voice as a Nurse—One Shift at a Time

Stephanee Beggs, MSN, RN

Debrief

True Stories of Advocating for Patients, Building Resilience, and Finding Your Voice as a Nurse—One Shift at a Time

For more information: steph@nursesteph.com
ISBN eBook: 978-1-962280-98-3
ISBN Paperback: 978-1-962280-99-0
ISBN Hardcover: 978-1-968164-00-3

For Momma B,
You're my "why."

Dear You,

"Are you writing it down to remember it or to forget it?" someone once asked, glancing at the pages of my red journal, filled with hurried scribbles and unfinished thoughts.

Stories from the emergency department (ED)—of life and loss, of victories so small they barely made a ripple, and failures so heavy they threatened to pull me under. The mistakes I've made. The patients I've held on to—and the ones I've had to let go. The lessons that took years to sink in. The moments that have shaped me into the nurse I am today.

"I write it down so I can feel it—and so I no longer have to carry it," I replied.

Which is true. But it wasn't always.

When I was a new nurse, I wrote things down to forget. To push past the weight of what I wasn't ready to face—the doubt that crept in after a tough shift, the exhaustion that settled into my bones, the heartbreak of realizing that sometimes, doing everything right still isn't enough. But now, as I return to these pages, I see something else.

Growth.

Perspective.

The proof that I was never standing still. I was always learning, always becoming.

So I debrief now, on these pages, for you.

For the moments when you feel like you're drowning.

For the nights when you wonder if you'll ever feel confident.

For the days when the weight of this profession feels unbearable.

You are not alone.

With love,
Nurse Steph

Table Of Contents

Introduction

No matter what you face in nursing, I hope you hold onto your good heart. The stories that stay with you, the words that break your silence, the moments that leave you changed—they shape you in quiet ways. But don't let them harden you. Let them remind you of the kind of nurse you promised yourself you'd be: present, kind, and still deeply human.

—Anonymous

"Nursing is *exactly* where I'm supposed to be."

This realization was a welcome one, though I arrived at it under the worst circumstances. My mother was unexpectedly diagnosed with stage 4 cholangiocarcinoma—a rare and aggressive form of gallbladder cancer that accounts for just 2 percent of global cancer diagnoses, with a five-year survival rate of only 3 percent. Overnight, I became not just her daughter but her caregiver.

While devastating, the role itself wasn't unfamiliar. In fact, I had just returned to school to pursue nursing when her diagnosis came. Before that, I'd earned a degree in business marketing—what felt like a natural fit for someone raised in a family of entrepreneurs.

Some of my earliest and fondest memories are of sitting with my siblings in the living room, watching Oprah at 3 p.m. while the aroma of my mother's latest kitchen creation filled the air. And every afternoon, at 3:05, my father would return home from the office and recount every detail of his day to her. We would listen, only half engaged, our attention split between the conversation and the comfort of routine. Business was the language of our household.

My mother was a powerhouse CEO, launching a software company from the garage of our small Burbank home in the nineties and eventually selling her first piece of software to Microsoft. That deal catapulted the business into success. My father? He served as the company's president, working under her leadership in the office. How badass is that?

My siblings followed suit. My sister built a thriving career in graphic design, which took her from New York to Northern California before she eventually launched a brand of her own. My brother carved out a career in the film industry—, starting with our high school football team and eventually editing for Netflix and HBO through his own postproduction firm.

And then there was me.

Every family has the one who doesn't quite follow the script … Hi, I'm Steph. I'll own my rebellious streak; those teenage years were something else. When it came time for college, I chose business marketing by default, stepping onto a structured, responsible path—one that felt like the logical next step.

Still, something never quite fit. As I worked my way through Corporate America, I realized that what I had mistaken for my passion was merely familiarity. I wasn't *called* to business; I was comfortable with it. What I truly wanted was something different, something that felt more meaningful. That's when I turned to medicine.

To this day, people ask me if my mom's illness is what made me want to become a nurse. I always say no—I knew long before. But caring for her? That's what made me *certain*. It didn't ignite the flame, but it fanned it into something I could no longer ignore.

She passed away on a dreary Sunday in November 2019, midway through my nursing program, just before finals week and the start of winter break. It's poignant, really. That semester, I was immersed in my labor and delivery and pediatrics rotations—two areas she had always been especially eager to hear about. She loved listening to my nursing school stories, but what excited her most were the ones about babies and children. When her illness required overnight hospital stays, I would take her on "field trips," gently wheeling her to the obstetrics (OB) floor so we could peer into the nursery together. One of her many hospitalizations remains etched in my memory. Admitted for jaundice, she stayed overnight for observation. I had just finished a pediatric clinical day at one hospital and drove to another to be with her. There she was, lying in her hospital bed, wearing her favorite panda shirt, while I sat beside her in my nursing school scrubs. We talked for hours, connected by a shared curiosity, both of us finding joy in learning and exploring new things, no matter the topic. I told her about my hectic day at clinical, and she responded with a flurry of questions about the patients' conditions and the care I had provided. At times, I wondered if she was truly fascinated by it all or if she simply found joy in seeing my enthusiasm for the work. Regardless, I'll never forget the smile on her face as she listened to my stories, even as she fought her own physical struggles.

In the final week of her life, her health deteriorated rapidly. She lost the strength to speak or move, and her days became a continuous stretch of sleep, interrupted only by fleeting moments of awareness when she would softly mention birds and butterflies in the sky. She had transformed into a shadow of the vibrant woman she once was—frail, unrecognizable, her body weakened, her hair thinned.

Amid this, I still had clinicals to complete: one last day of OB rotations and one final exam before winter break. I sat beside her, the sound of her death rattle almost a constant hum in the room, as I studied. The soft strains of gospel music filled the air, a calming contrast to the heaviness that enveloped us both. On the seventh day of her decline, she took her final breath. I listened with my stethoscope, feeling the weight of the silence that followed, and held her cold, lifeless hands in mine. With the hospice nurse, I gently changed her into her favorite pajamas. And when the time came, I helped transfer her into a body bag—a final act of care before she was taken from the home where she had raised me.

Although my professor had told me I didn't need to attend my final clinical day—especially after having just zipped my own mother into a body bag the day before—I went anyway. My heart was shattered, but I knew I had to keep moving.

I was assigned to the operating room (OR) for a twin cesarean section. However, my instructor pulled me from the OR and insisted I spend the entire twelve-hour shift in the newborn nursery instead. And so that's where I went. I spent the day holding, rocking, and feeding newborns with the nurses in a small, twelve-by-twelve room, bassinets lining the walls, with soft music playing from a nurse's cell phone in the background. "Dance Monkey" played on repeat for nearly half the day. It was her favorite song, she said, and little did she know, it became mine as well—not for the song itself but for the memory it gave me. A moment I hadn't even realized I needed.

As I reflect on that day years later, I realize something extraordinary. In the span of twenty-four hours, I lived through both life and death—two forces so starkly contrasting yet inseparable. How beautifully unique it is to witness such opposing spectrums. I stood at the threshold of both the beginning and the end, and in the still, fragile space between, I discovered a well of strength within myself. Some people wonder why I still went to clinical the next day. The experience was undeniably traumatic, yet I understood that life, in all its complexity, would continue. People were still counting on me. It is this understanding—this quiet resilience—that has shaped my path and, perhaps, is why I find myself so deeply drawn to emergency medicine.

The ability to compartmentalize and move forward in the face of trauma is the silent power that sustains a nurse.

Since that day, life has unfolded in ways I never could have imagined. It's been a remarkable journey: graduating from nursing school the same month a global pandemic was declared, taking the National Council Licensure Examination (NCLEX) amid lockdowns, and beginning my dream career in the emergency department. Most unexpected of all was the creation of RNExplained, a nationally recognized educational platform aimed at supporting and educating nursing students and registered nurses globally. What started as a simple way to share study tips online has since evolved tenfold, reaching millions and evolving into a community with purpose, connection, and impact.

But let's back up for a moment. I'm in a great place now, and I truly find joy in sharing resources and education with my community. (If you're reading this, that community includes you. Welcome!) If you know me, you know that I believe every experience holds a lesson, and I'll *always* find a way to turn a moment into an opportunity for learning.

Your grandma fell in the living room? Let's talk about environmental fall risk factors and the signs of shortening. Witness a motor vehicle accident (MVA) and you're the only one there? Let me show you how to critically assess potential worst-case scenarios and how to respond effectively before emergency medical services (EMS) arrives. My mom died in front of my eyes? I'll teach you about the death rattle and postmortem care. You get the idea—I'm a sucker for a teaching moment, no matter how happy, tragic, or messy the story may be.

But getting here? It wasn't exactly conventional.

After I realized that business marketing wasn't filling my cup (more like draining it), I knew I needed to find a path that truly meshed with my passions and skills. And as any postcollege graduate facing an identity crisis would, I dove headfirst into a full-blown mental spiral of *Wait, what* am *I actually good at?* As a child, I'd always been fascinated by the medical field, often imagining myself as an anesthesiologist, captivated by the idea of working in a hospital. At that young age, though, I hadn't yet grasped the full range of opportunities within the world of medicine.

Eventually, I found my calling in nursing—a decision that, in hindsight, feels entirely natural. With my innate sense of care and a strong aptitude for science, math, and anatomy, I quickly realized that nursing was where my strengths intersected. So without hesitation, I dove in.

What I hadn't fully anticipated, however, was the solitude of navigating this new path. Without any family or friends with medical backgrounds to guide me, it felt like I was diving into uncharted waters without a map. On my days off, I immersed myself in researching nursing programs, exploring every option, prerequisite, application deadline, and strategy to be competitive. Every decision I made—every step, every choice—was my own, crafted through hours of diligent self-study, with no outside counsel.

I won't sugarcoat it—doubt often crept in. I feared my parents would disapprove of such a dramatic change in direction. The weight of disappointment—the feeling of "starting over"—was heavier than I anticipated. At twenty-three, returning to school felt like I was back at square one. *Four years of college, for what?* The fear of judgment—*What will people think?*—lingered at the back of my mind, especially after I had already invested so much time earning a business degree, only to set it aside. It was a mental shift that frequently had me questioning whether I was making the right choice.

Nevertheless, I trusted my gut and applied to schools offering accelerated bachelor of science in nursing (ABSN) programs. With my prior bachelor's degree, I qualified for these rigorous paths, which allowed me to bypass general education courses I had already completed and jump straight into the nursing core and clinical rotations. They always say, "You've got to be a little crazy to take on an accelerated program." And they aren't wrong. Twelve months of relentless coursework and clinical rotations—six days a week, ten to twelve hours a day. No bullshit. No fluff. Just done. Career path solidified.

It was time to get to work, literally and figuratively. I took on four jobs and volunteer positions while juggling a full course load of science prerequisites—classes I hadn't needed as a business major but now had to complete for nursing school admissions. After class on weekdays, I worked as a server (a role that admissions departments highly value, by the way) and volunteered at the nation's #1 hospital—the same hospital my mom had spent many nights during her illness. On weekend mornings, I worked as a medical scribe in an ER-based urgent care, and on weekend evenings, I volunteered at a senior center (a job I didn't love but knew would boost my nursing school application). If "hustle" had a name, it would have been mine.

After enduring a string of rejections—five in total, including one particularly disheartening denial from my alma mater—I will never forget the moment I finally received what I had worked so tirelessly toward: an acceptance letter from Mount Saint Mary's University. The flood of emotions was overwhelming: relief, excitement, anticipation, a hint of anxiety about what the future held, and above all, a profound sense of pride. Without hesitation, I called my parents, eager to share the news.

"Mom! Dad!" I shouted into the phone, breathless with excitement. "I got into nursing school!"

"Wh-what?" came the faint reply.

"I got into nursing school!" I yelled again, louder this time.

"What? We can't hear yo—"

And then, silence. The plane they were on had just taken off and, with it, my big moment. The connection was lost, and I wouldn't be able to share the news until hours later, when they finally landed.

I couldn't help but laugh to myself. *Of course.* The one time I finally had big news, the call dropped. It played out like a movie scene.

If you're reading this, you know nursing school felt like the longest marathon ever—yet somehow, life has a way of speeding by. Six months after that call, I'd wave goodbye to any semblance of a social life and dive headfirst into an exhausting schedule of classrooms, clinicals, and exams, six days a week. Just six months after that, my mom would be gone, and six months after that, I'd be graduating during a global pandemic—no pinning ceremony, no celebrations. Two months later, I'd pass my boards, earn my license, and step straight into the ER, which, as you probably guessed, was where I always wanted to be. A timeline so unconventional yet a raw and beautiful portrait of resilience.

The timing of this book's release was no accident; it was published on the five-year anniversary of my officially becoming a nurse—when I finally earned those two letters behind my name and began a journey that would profoundly change me.

I invite you to experience the nursing profession through *my* lens—a raw collection of profound challenges and defining moments that have shaped me into the nurse I am today. From the demanding realities of new grad residency to navigating loss and bullying, to finding my voice in a field that often asks more than we can give, these stories reflect the moments that have left an indelible mark on me. The stories shared in this book are those that found a permanent place in my red journal—ones marked by a powerful lesson learned, a mistake made, or an experience that I couldn't quite shake, and in debriefing them with you, my hope is that you will find comfort and relatability too.

The concept of debriefing is vital to both professional growth and mental clarity, yet it is frequently dismissed to the background, overlooked in favor of an unyielding pace. In the relentless world of health care, where urgency and constant demands define every moment, debriefing becomes a luxury—one that the system too often disregards in the rush from task to task. Often, there's an unspoken expectation to push through without acknowledging the emotional toll. Yet that very pause—the space where we can reflect—is perhaps the most crucial part of the job.

Debrief is a call for reflection. When the system says, *We don't have time for that,* I'm here saying, *Take a moment to reflect, to learn.* I firmly believe that we are a collective of each other's victories and mistakes, and by embracing both—by reflecting on both—we can grow together as nurses. So what better way to debrief than by starting with my own experiences—pouring out my heart, sharing my lessons, and offering what I've learned along the way?

Let's get started.

Baptism by Fire

I graduated from nursing school in April 2020—one month after the World Health Organization (WHO) declared COVID-19 a pandemic. By the end of that month, more than half a million people had been infected, and nearly thirty thousand had died. In the coming years, it would become one of the deadliest global health crises in modern history, reshaping the world—and the health care field—in ways we're still trying to understand.

Lockdowns were in full effect, hospitals were at capacity, and I—little ole fresh new grad nurse Stephanee—was stepping into the profession at a time when the need for nurses had never been more urgent.

Before I walked across that (virtual) stage, my last nursing instructor sent me an email:

"It was an honor to have you in my class. Welcome to the world of nursing—now hurry up, because we need you."

Or so I thought.

I applied to seven different new graduate programs across Southern California. *Seven*. And I was rejected from all but one.

How could that be? Amid a global pandemic—when hospitals were desperate for more health care workers—why wouldn't they hire ... *me?*

I later learned that, because of the overwhelming demand during a pandemic, hospitals preferred nurses who were already trained. It was easier to bring someone out of retirement than to invest the time and money required to get a new grad up to speed.

In the end, though, it worked in my favor—I landed exactly where I wanted to be, in the unit I had dreamed of since the beginning of nursing school: the emergency department.

Out of two thousand applicants for the ER, only two of us were hired. And of all the units to be placed in during a crisis of this scale, the ER—along with critical care and other frontline units—was one of the most intense, unpredictable, and frankly, terrifying places to be.

But I didn't feel scared walking into the unknown. I felt ready—ready to work, ready to learn, ready to do whatever I could to help. My attitude wasn't *Oh no, it's a pandemic. I'm scared of catching COVID or seeing death.* It was *Just put me in. Let's go. Let's learn.*

I don't have any frame of reference for what nursing was like before COVID. To this day, when anyone asks me what it was like to be a nurse during the pandemic, I always respond, "That was my normal. That's all I knew nursing to be." And it's true! I didn't know any different.

Years later, when things finally started to calm down, my coworkers would say, "We're almost back to what it used to be pre-COVID." But I will *never* truly understand what that felt like. A crisis became my normal. Swabbing every single patient, regardless of respiratory symptoms, became my normal. N95s, head-to-toe PPE, and shouting over maxed-out high-flow machines became my normal.

In many ways, beginning my nursing career amid the worst of the worst was a peculiar blessing. Having navigated through a global health crisis and witnessed things I never imagined I would, I've learned that few things in this field can truly faze me anymore. It's a feeling I hadn't experienced since the day my mom passed, when I bagged her body with my own two hands. It's as if the universe threw me into the fire, and now, the flames don't seem as hot.

But I want to walk you through some of the experiences that marked this time: conditions we worked in, patients who still linger in my mind, and feelings I can't quite shake. Because while some of you reading this may relate to those chaotic, uncertain moments, others may never have had to experience it. And to that, I say, *Thank God*. Still, it's important for me to show you where I came from, to give you a glimpse into what shaped me and the kind of nurse I became through it all.

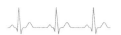

The environment we worked in was far from what I had envisioned or was accustomed to from my nursing school training, and it quickly became evident that no amount of preparation could fully equip me for the challenges ahead. The layout of the ER felt like a labyrinth, a mere shadow of its former state, as I was told.

"These are our COVID isolation rooms," a nurse said, gesturing to the bright-red tape that outlined the doorframes of what would otherwise be standard isolation rooms. The doors had been replaced with plastic tarps, with small clear windows offering a bird's-eye view into the rooms. It was one of the *few* things I had seen depicted in TV shows that was spot-on, capturing the grim communication between nurse and patient through a plastic barrier. Inside, a gurney (or two) were stationed, and the loud hum of a high-efficiency particulate air (HEPA) filter filled the air—the hospital's best defense against dangerous airborne microbes.

I noticed one of the rooms was empty, a sign with a circle-backslash symbol hanging on the door. I glanced at it, puzzled.

"EVS [Environmental Services] has to come by to sterilize this one," the nurse explained. "We call it a 'terminal' clean."

Terminal? Did the patient die?

"Whenever a COVID-positive patient is discharged, admitted, or expires, the room must be thoroughly sterilized and left empty for at least thirty minutes with the HEPA filter running. It helps clear out any lingering virus in the air. It's protocol—we can't just flip the room like we normally would."

I nodded, taking in all the new terminology and information.

She led me to another area. "And over here, we turned the manager's office into another COVID area, but this is for patients who don't need to be on a monitor—like ones with mild shortness of breath or just aches and pains." She pointed to a cramped room the size of a small closet. Inside were three gurneys, a chair, and mobile vital signs machines. The room felt stuffy, almost suffocating—an ideal breeding ground for COVID. But there appeared to be no other option.

"Then we have our regular rooms over here for non-COVID complaints. But don't be surprised if you get a patient with vaginal bleeding, and when you swab, they test positive for COVID. It's fair game in here now; we try to keep the COVID and non-COVID patients separate, but at this point, it's impossible to separate them completely." She motioned to the back end of the department, where gurneys were separated only by curtains. Duct-taped signs marked each one with a "+" to indicate a positive COVID result. It was clear they had done their best to keep the two groups apart, but with COVID running rampant, the virus was inescapable—even in the least expected patients.

She walked me down to the farthest corner of the unit, where the hallway seemed to dead-end in a cramped space.

"This room here," she said, pointing, "used to be triage. Now, it's just another makeshift area for more gurneys. Triage is outside now, but don't worry—we're getting there." The space, no bigger than a small bathroom, now held four more gurneys.

We stepped outside into what I could only describe as a war zone—in every sense of the word. The emergency department had spilled into the parking garage, where massive sandbags lined the perimeter of the first floor, a desperate attempt to keep the rain from flooding the makeshift treatment area. Large white tents stretched across parking spaces, forming an impromptu nurses' station outfitted with three computers, desks, workstations on wheels (WOWs), a Pyxis stocked with a limited selection of medications, and a so-called supply room—a single table cluttered with bins of haphazardly gathered supplies from inside.

A long tarped tunnel served as the patient care area. Inside, gurneys were crammed together, separated by thin metal privacy screens—or sometimes, nothing at all. The space was illuminated by hanging LED work lights, the kind used in construction zones for overnight highway repairs. In one section, chairs formed a designated area for "fast-track" patients—those needing medication refills, minor wound care, or something as trivial as a stubbed toe. Because even in the midst of a global pandemic, the ER doors remained open to all.

Triage had also been relocated here. Hospital couches—dragged from inside—were now lined up in the parking lot, where patients sat waiting to be assessed. A small white tent functioned as the triage space, manned by one or two nurses and an EMT. Patients were quickly evaluated, entered into the system, and depending on the severity of their symptoms, either wheeled inside by an EMT to be bedded in the main ER or left outside to wait.

And that's how we operated—on plastic tarps, without air conditioning or heat in winter. PPE shortages forced us to rewear the same N95 mask all day long, its straps digging into our skin, leaving behind marks that never seemed to fade.

I did as much of my assessment as I could from outside the room, peering through the plastic window to check vital signs or watch my patient's work of breathing from afar—like they were a caged animal at the zoo. And truthfully, that's exactly how it felt.

Patients would yell out requests, their voices muffled by layers of plastic, oxygen masks, and distance, and I'd shout back from the other side of the barrier. We tried to keep our distance for our own safety, but when it came down to it, we were right up in the exhibit—intubating, turning, performing CPR—drowning in the very air we feared.

And when I finally got to my car in the parking lot after a shift, I would sit in silence, gripping the steering wheel, replaying everything I had just endured. No music, no podcasts—just the hum of the engine and the deserted roads stretching emptily ahead.

At home, I stripped down at the doorstep, peeling off each layer like contaminated skin. Straight into the wash. Then a scorching shower.

Go to bed. Get up. Do it all over again the next day.

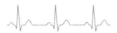

The emergency department where I work treats both adults and pediatric patients, as do most hospitals that are not specifically designated as pediatric-only facilities. This was not something that changed during the pandemic. While COVID-like symptoms became the prevailing "it girl" complaint at the time, the patients we saw remained diverse in age. Some were children, others were young adults in their twenties, but the majority were older adults—many of whom had comorbidities that put them at far greater risk.

The first COVID-positive patient under my care was an older man in his seventies. I remember him vividly—he sat in Room 8 at the edge of the bed in tripod position, his work of breathing noticeably exaggerated. It was also the first time I had ever fully gowned up. His COVID test result hadn't come back yet, but his symptoms and physical presentation practically screamed positive.

As I stood outside the doorway, tying my gown and securing my gloves in place, the physician assigned to his care walked up behind me. We had only worked together once before, but I remembered her well. She was a total badass—

intimidating by nature, with a direct and no-nonsense attitude. But what else did you expect in emergency medicine, especially in the middle of a pandemic?

"You're going in there, right?" she asked, pulling a gown from the shelf and draping it over herself.

"Yes, I am," I replied, eager and excited—still a fresh baby nurse.

"Okay, great. I'm coming too."

Okay! I thought to myself. I had dreamed of moments like this—working alongside the physician, putting our brains together to collaborate on the patients who needed us most.

She unzipped the plastic tarp that served as a barrier between us and him, stepping inside. I followed close behind.

"Hi, Mr. B, my name is Dr. Stevens. How are you feeling?" she asked, her voice slightly louder than usual, trying to be heard through the three layers of masks covering her mouth.

"I'm doing all right," he said, pausing between words to catch his breath. "I feel a little short of breath, but otherwise, I'm okay."

You could tell he was downplaying his symptoms, holding onto a glimmer of hope despite the unknown. He smiled, but I knew that smile was masking his fear.

Dr. Stevens cut right to the chase—no bullshit. "We got your results back, and you're positive for COVID."

She paused, giving him a moment to process the news. I sat in silence, allowing him the space to take it in.

"So we're going to keep you here in the hospital," she said. "And I want you to call your family, okay? I'm going to be honest—I'm not sure if you'll be leaving the hospital after this. Your chest X-ray looks nasty."

The expression on Mr. B's face was one of pure shock, as though he had just been handed a death sentence with no way to escape it. And to be honest, that's exactly what it was. What had started as a simple visit to the hospital for a COVID test had suddenly become a moment that would, for him, likely be the last. He didn't have the words to respond; how could he? Some moments are so immense that language fails entirely. There was no panic in his eyes—no outburst of emotion—just the heavy, oppressive weight of knowing that his world had just shifted irreversibly.

I felt a sudden heaviness in my chest, my stomach sinking—not for the reason you might think. Not because of the death sentence itself but because of the way it was delivered. I had never been in this position before—this moment was new, terrifying, and unbearably real. I had never witnessed someone being told, so bluntly, that they were going to die. Not in theory, not in a classroom discussion, but in real life—to a real person with a wife, kids, and grandkids.

So how do you say it *right*? *Is* there a right way? How do you even begin a conversation like that? You could soften the blow, sugarcoat it, ease them into the reality with carefully chosen words. Or you could rip the Band-Aid off and say it straight. A part of me wonders if the latter is just as much for us as it is for them—to protect *ourselves* from the weight of it, to create some distance from the truth.

Around us, the chaos of the ER continued—machines beeped, voices rose and fell, the hospital's steady pulse pressing on. Yet in that room, time felt suspended. I stood there, feeling a profound disconnect—not from the patient but from myself. My body was present, but my mind and soul felt distant, struggling to grasp the weight of this moment, the reality of this pandemic.

That was the sharpest realization of all: Sometimes, in the face of such overwhelming truth, all we can do is stand there, powerless.

This was my first real encounter with the virus—the first time it transcended the images on the news and became something deeply personal, something that demanded my attention in a way I hadn't expected. Until that moment, I had only understood COVID intellectually, through the lens of numbers and statistics, through the general hum of hospital life. But when Dr. Stevens uttered those words, so blunt and final—"You won't leave this hospital. Call your family."—I felt the magnitude of it. This was no longer a distant threat. It was immediate. It was real. And it was standing right in front of me.

Mr. B never made it out of that hospital. I couldn't help but wonder, did his family ever get to say a proper goodbye? Or was their final farewell through an iPad screen, like so many others in those early days? He became part of the statistic, one of countless lives claimed by the virus. But to me, he marked a turning point. He was the one who forced me to confront the depth of this crisis—reminding me that our profession asks us to bear witness to the things the outside world seldom sees.

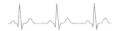

One particular day, I walked the familiar halls of the main emergency room, carrying out my typical duties. Though I was assigned to the non-COVID rooms, as mentioned earlier, the lines between these spaces often blurred, making it nearly impossible to contain the virus. As I moved down the hallway, I noticed a young girl sitting alone on a gurney, her face a mixture of fear and sadness. She looked around, perhaps searching for a familiar face, but I saw no guardian with her.

I approached and introduced myself. "Hi, my name is Stephanee, and I'll be your nurse today. What brings you in?" Her response, spoken in a tone heavy with defeat, immediately stopped me in my tracks: "I don't want to live anymore. I'm so tired of this."

I had not reviewed her chart before our conversation, so her words took me by surprise. Without hesitation, I sat on the edge of her bed, meeting her eye level. "What makes you say that?" I asked, my voice gentle.

The girl, just fourteen years old and a freshman in high school, had attempted suicide by ingesting a handful of over-the-counter Tylenol. As a nurse, I knew that this amount likely wouldn't be fatal, but to her, it seemed like the only escape. She told me that, after the transition to online schooling, she found herself staring at her own face on a screen for hours each day. Over time, this constant exposure to her reflection began to fuel intense self-loathing. She hated the way she looked, the sound of her laugh, even the quick glimpses of her face during Zoom classes. Eventually, this deep self-rejection became so overwhelming that she believed the only way to escape herself was through death.

And that's something I feel is often overlooked—the unseen impact of COVID. While the headlines focused on the devastating toll it took on the elderly and immunocompromised, there were far-reaching consequences that extended well beyond just physical illness. For those of us on the front lines, it wasn't just about "treating the virus"; we also had to pick up the pieces of lives shattered by the pandemic in ways that didn't always make the news. Increased rates of homelessness, job loss, isolation, and in particular, a surge in mental health issues—issues that affected people much younger than most would ever expect. Because when individuals face a crisis, regardless of its nature, where do they turn? The emergency department. And what do we do? We never turn them away.

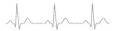

Starting my career during this time taught me many lessons—some expected, like the value of teamwork and the importance of appreciating life. But in retrospect, this unique combination revealed far deeper realities about this profession and the world around me.

Trust the experts—but recognize that not everyone who speaks is one. In this country and throughout our health care system, we are fortunate to have some of the most knowledgeable and dedicated professionals who worked tirelessly to combat the COVID-19 crisis. Yet it was deeply concerning to see social media and public figures challenge basic science, spreading misinformation with potentially harmful consequences.

One of the most egregious examples came when President Donald Trump suggested that injecting bleach might be a potential solution to COVID-19. As absurd as it sounded, the true danger wasn't just the statement itself but the fact that people believed it.

I remember one patient—a man in his early thirties—who, in an act of desperation and perhaps influenced by this rhetoric, drank bleach in an attempt to fight the virus. I passed by his room one day, instinctively glancing through the plastic window, as I always did. What I saw still haunts me. His face was barely recognizable, his eyes, cheeks, and lips eroded beyond recognition, with only an endotracheal tube protruding from his mouth. The damage was catastrophic. He was slowly bleeding out internally, his body destroyed by what he had ingested. We kept him on a ventilator for a day or two, but there was no way to save him.

You cannot live in crisis mode forever—at some point, normal must be redefined. This realization was deeply personal for me. In the years following the pandemic, I had to unlearn the survival-driven mindset that had shaped my early experiences in nursing. Early on, my actions were guided by crisis protocols, rapid interventions, and constant adaptation to evolving news. But as the immediate threat subsided, I had to recalibrate—learning how to provide care in a world no longer defined by survival mode.

The challenge wasn't just adjusting my approach to patient care; it was rewiring my instincts and rediscovering what it meant to be a nurse beyond the context of a global emergency.

Care for the caregiver. While the news hailed us as heroes and we got discounts from local businesses and praise from our neighbors, the reality often felt different. The recognition, though appreciated, wasn't enough to counterbalance the heavy toll on our own health. Shit, I had seventeen coworkers quit or transfer to other hospitals in a two-month span, which left me—just a few months into the job—as one of the most "senior" staff members. When I caught COVID myself, the only message I recieved was "When are you cleared to come back?" What does that say about management and working conditions? We worked long hours beyond the standard twelve-hour shifts, our units were constantly short-staffed, and the patient load kept growing.

For me, this was a sobering reminder of why we're here: for our patients. My existence as an employee often felt reduced to that alone, and it reinforced the critical importance of taking care of myself—physically and emotionally. Because at the end of the day, the only person who will look after you … is you. I like to think I'm fully recovered from COVID, but every time I put on an N95, the smell and claustrophobia take me right back to that time. Every time I see a patient struggling with a bilevel positive airway pressure (BiPAP), gasping for air and begging not to die, I'm back again.

Initiation Day

I never imagined my career would lead me here—on my hands and knees, chasing maggots across the floor with a pair of tweezers. It wasn't exactly the heroic image I had when I first entered this profession, but there I was, living it.

But let's back up. One cold January, EMS brought in a patient without prior warning or phone call, which is rare. Nine times out of ten, they call ahead, giving a heads-up on the situation and their estimated time of arrival. But every so often, they show up unannounced, and in my experience, it's almost always with patients from specific populations: those experiencing homelessness or individuals in custody needing medical clearance, for example.

Medics wheeled in the patient, who was experiencing homelessness. Outwardly, he was extremely dirty and carried a strong smell of old mildew—so strong I considered doubling up my masks.

> Pro tip: For patients with overwhelming odors (Clostridioides difficile [C. diff], gastrointestinal [GI bleed], poor hygiene), grab some toothpaste from the supply room or a roll-on essential oil (I swear by peppermint from Amazon) and put a generous amount between two masks. Boom—no more gagging.

Because he was so unkempt, I couldn't get an accurate sense of his age. He looked like he could be in his seventies, but he might have only been in his fifties.

As the ER staff, it was our job to figure out why he was there. According to the medics, a bystander had called 911, concerned that he might be having a serious medical issue due to his slurred speech. Upon their own assessment, they confirmed that he was indeed slurring his words and struggling to communicate. It wasn't immediately clear whether he might be intoxicated, had a naturally low baseline for communication, or something more serious was going on. But regardless of his appearance or living situation, he deserved a thorough evaluation—just like any other patient.

There are only a few isolation rooms in the ER reserved for infectious patients—tuberculosis, respiratory syncytial virus (RSV), C. diff—or for procedures requiring privacy, like pelvic ultrasounds. Occasionally, in desperate moments, we use them to contain overpowering odors. That day, my assignment included one isolation room … and that's where this patient ended up. Our physician tried to ask him the standard questions: Where do you live? Have you had anything to drink? Do you have any pain? But the patient didn't seem to have the capacity to answer. After a few failed attempts, the doctor sighed, rolled his eyes in a silent *Why are you even here if you're not going to talk?* and told me to get him cleaned up, saying he'd plan to loop back later. I interpreted that decision as putting less priority on this patient because of his appearance, but I was a new grad— only four months into the job—and did what I was told.

I've always been observant—keenly aware of shifts in tone, subtle changes in facial expressions, who favors whom, who dismisses whom. I notice the unspoken judgments, the quiet ways care shifts based on personal bias. Maybe it comes from my own experiences. Growing up, I was constantly judged for things beyond my control. I had to fight for respect in every accomplishment I earned—maybe because I was a woman in a male-dominated field? Maybe because of my hair color, or because I looked too young? People made assumptions, dismissed me before they ever got to know me.

And as a new grad, I faced similar challenges. Coworkers dismissed me from the start. (We're friends now, so yes— there was light at the end of the tunnel.) At the time, there was no clear reason for the tension, and later, when we finally connected, they admitted their initial judgments had no real basis.

I was talked about. People made comments about me and the success of my business. They judged my work ethic and my desire to work in the ER based on nothing more than a few twenty-second interactions. I had to work twice as hard to earn the respect that should have been there from the start—from the very people I had worked so hard to stand beside. And let me tell you, that kind of experience takes a toll on your mental health. It chips away at your confidence, shifts the way you see yourself, and forces you to become hyperaware of how people treat others. But it also reshapes your compassion. It makes you more empathetic, more determined not to let anyone feel the way you did. That's why, no matter what I think or feel, I refuse to let my own biases—or anyone else's—affect the care I give.

The gentleman in front of me that day was so soiled that I had to take my trauma shears and start cutting away at his socks. The cold and rainy weather had left the wet dirt hardened, molding the fabric to his feet. His shoes had disintegrated into fragments, barely holding together. The smell lingered in the halls, drawing the attention of other nurses. Experienced staff popped in, not to help, but to gawk, laugh, and carry gossip back to the nurses' station about his stench and appearance.

"Don't worry," I told him. "I'm going to clean you up."

I cut through the calf-high socks, and as I peeled the first one away from his skin, maggots swarmed his leg—so many that I couldn't even see his skin beneath them. Hundreds, if not thousands, of tiny white bugs wriggled over each other, spilling out from the fabric. They tumbled onto the floor, onto the gurney, onto my hands.

He didn't react. He didn't even seem to notice they were there. They'd clearly been there for a while, attracted by the moisture and the infected abrasions scattered along his lower shin and ankle.

My knee-jerk reaction was to back away. I'd never seen anything like this. Sure, I'd passed homeless people on the street, but I had never interacted with one in this capacity.

Then came the confusion. *What the hell am I supposed to do?* As a brand-new nurse, I had no idea how to troubleshoot this or what the proper protocol was. *Shit, is there even a protocol for this??*

Today, I actually love running into challenging problems like this. I know that once I figure out a solution and learn all the resources available, it will help me serve the next patient better. But back then, I didn't have the tools or experience. So I told him I needed to step out for a minute and went to ask the other nurses for guidance. When I explained what I had found, they smirked. "Well, you have to clean the maggots out. That's your initiation. Welcome to the ER."

Out of all the moments when I had witnessed the negative effects of being jaded, *this* one hit differently. It made my personal experiences resurface—the times I'd been dismissed, underestimated, or made to prove myself for no reason other than seniority demanding it.

At the end of the day, I have nothing but love for my coworkers. But in that moment, I felt the weight of their indifference. I saw the line between experience and cynicism, between resilience and detachment. And I knew, without a doubt, that I never wanted to cross it.

My preceptor took care of our other three patients so I could focus solely on this one. It was toward the end of my preceptorship, and my main priorities had shifted to troubleshooting situations where I had no idea what to do. Who could I turn to when I was "alone" and unsure? What ideas could I come up with on my own in the meantime? How could I delegate care for other patients who needed me while I was tied up with this one? His condition wasn't life-threateningly critical, but my preceptor wanted me to get exposure to the problem-solving side of nursing, and I respected her for helping me see the bigger picture. So I turned to her for guidance, and after a quick evaluation, she suggested using hydrogen peroxide to get the maggots off.

I completely gowned up—head to toe. Eyewear, gown, double gloves, double masks, booties. I went into the medication room to grab a few bottles of hydrogen peroxide, then gathered a large basin, towels, and a few red biohazard bags. Returning to the room, I had him scoot to the edge of the bed so his legs dangled off. As ER nurses, we're used to improvising and creating makeshift workspaces, so I used the red biohazard bags to form a temporary basin around the bed, draping them from each corner to catch the maggots and keep the area contained. For the next two hours, I poured hydrogen peroxide over his legs, watching as the maggots fell off in clumps, tumbling into my makeshift basin. Every so often, a few would escape and crawl across the floor, so tweezers became my best friend as I picked up the remaining stragglers.

The process allowed me ample time to get to know him beyond first impressions. Despite his outward appearance, he was kind—gentle, even. It was clear that few had ever taken the time to truly see him. He shared that he'd fallen on hard times and now called the highway overpass "home." His speech was mumbled and, at times, difficult to understand, but that alone wasn't reason enough for EMS to bring him in. Thankfully, they did—because while he needed treatment, he was also due for someone to simply listen.

When I finished, I handed him what we call "purple wipes"—thick antibacterial adult bath wipes—and gave him space to clean the rest of his body. I tossed his mildewed clothes and brought him fresh ones, along with a turkey sandwich and some water. We spent time together, and I believe he seemed to experience something beyond just the bare minimum care.

Once we were done, the physician came back to reassess him. Unfortunately, the visit didn't lead to much else—he was quickly discharged without further intervention. I called in social work, gathered local homeless resources, and made sure he left with extra food and water.

That experience stayed with me—for many reasons. Some were deeply personal, tied to this stranger and the man he was. Others surfaced when I stepped back and considered the broader picture, the systems and assumptions that shaped our encounter.

I come from privilege. I grew up with a strong support system, access to education, and a life that kept me far from the margins. That privilege carries responsibility—to recognize it, stay grounded in reality, and never allow it to distort how I see others.

Growing up, my mother often said, "You're as good as anybody. But never forget you're no better than anybody, either." She drilled those words into our heads. And there I was—standing in a room with a man twice my age, soiled in dirt, as I held a biohazard bag full of maggots—face to face with the rawest version of her lesson. I had a choice: to let my privilege cloud my view of someone who, on the surface, seemed lesser…or to see him fully. Not as a diagnosis or a list of symptoms, but as a human being. And to meet him not with judgment, but with dignity and compassion.

Looking back, some called it an *initiation*—a rite of passage into the chaos of emergency medicine. They laughed, they gawked, and then they moved on. But I didn't. I felt the weight of their indifference, heavy and undeniable. I learned that treating someone with dignity isn't just a sentiment; it's a discipline. It's a choice you make even when you're overwhelmingly busy, when the room is filled with maggots, or when no one else seems to care. It's what separates the task of nursing from the heart of it. And although emergency medicine is notorious for its hardheaded personalities, I knew it was important to be the kind of nurse who never lets that intensity erase the humanity right in front of me.

That night, I sat in my bed (don't worry, I took a long, hot shower first) replaying the entire situation in my head. The concept of dignity lingered, and I realized it extended far beyond my patient. It was so much bigger than that. As always, I reached for my red journal, scribbling down two words: *care* and *caring*. They look nearly identical on the page, but in practice, they couldn't be more different. One is procedural; the other, personal.

To provide *care* means to check the boxes, follow the protocols, administer the treatments. It's what nursing school prepares us for—skills, systems, and evidence-based practice. But here's the unfortunate truth: Many people will become excellent at providing care while completely missing the human being sitting right in front of them. That's what happens when *caring* is absent.

Caring, on the other hand, demands presence. It asks you to pause, to listen, to notice the person beyond the chart or the diagnosis. And in emergency medicine—where the pace is unrelenting and the pressure is high—those two things can quietly drift apart.

The culture of the ER doesn't always make space for caring. We pride ourselves on being fast, efficient, and unshakable. Teamwork is critical, but it often revolves around logistics: Who's got the next trauma? Who's starting the IV? Who's running the code? Of course, those roles are essential. But I learned that *true* teamwork goes beyond task management—it includes emotional accountability. It means creating a space where slowing down to care doesn't make you weak or inefficient, but human.

That shift taught me the kind of nurse I want to be— not just someone who gets things done, but someone who sees people clearly, even when the system doesn't. I never want to lose sight of the fact that *care* is what the job demands, but *caring* is what the patient remembers. And honoring someone's dignity, even in the most undignified moments, is what gives this work meaning.

The Click

I find it fascinating that in nearly every situation in life, you're thrown all this information—rules, new people, expectations—and then one day, it just *clicks*. You find your way, and somehow, you *did* it.

I remember walking into the emergency department for the very first time, completely in awe of the job I had dreamed of since prerequisites. I left that day thinking, *Holy shit. Information overload. How am I possibly going to remember all of this and even compare to these badass nurses around me?*

On my first official day on the floor, I was given a patient in supraventricular tachycardia (SVT). The chaos around me—the chatter, the leads, the IV start, the EKG capture—still plays in my head like a movie. It was like I was a fly on the wall, watching it all unfold. But in reality, I was smack dab in the middle of it. Face-to-face with a real human patient. *My* patient.

Dr. B walked in, my first time ever speaking or working alongside a doctor as an official nurse. He evaluated the EKG, handed the patient an empty syringe, and said, "Take a deep breath and blow into this for fifteen seconds."

I stared, completely confused. He glanced at me and said, "Grab a leg."

Before I could process what was happening, my preceptor dropped the head of the bed while we flipped the patient's legs upside down. Head down, legs up. I looked at my preceptor in disbelief, thinking, *Where on Earth did I just get hired?*

After fifteen weeks of preceptorship, I felt like I knew *so much* and *nothing* at the same time. The policies, the procedures, the never-ending checklists—I was drowning in them. I would see a task and go completely blank, even if I had done it eighty times before. Shit, even three or four months into working on my own, I'd *still* spike the wrong end of an IV bag—despite spiking twenty IV bags a day.

I felt like a shell of myself, just going through the motions to survive the shift. I was so task oriented that I wasn't even sure who *I* was as a nurse. *Who was Stephanee as a nurse?*

But then—one day—it *clicked.*

The blinders slowly came off.

You kick fear, insecurity, and doubt to the curb, and you just *do the damn thing.*

Bridging the gap between textbook knowledge and real-world bedside practice is one of the biggest challenges in transitioning from student to nurse. In fact, I'd argue it's the steepest learning curve—and one of my biggest frustrations with nursing curricula. Nursing school teaches you to recognize jaundice and its possible origins, but it doesn't emphasize how alkaline phosphatase (ALP) helps differentiate hepatic from biliary causes. It drills standard protocols for choking but never mentions that Diet Coke and nitroglycerin can sometimes relieve an esophageal obstruction. Or that if a patient has a rectal prolapse, the doctor might send you to the cafeteria for sugar packets.

> *Nursing school presents a black-and-white version of patient care, but the real world exists in fifty shades of gray. It took me months before I finally had my ah-ha moment—before I truly understood not just what I was doing but why.*

I remember the exact moment it happened.

I was caring for a hypotensive patient, and instead of automatically following a protocol, I stepped back and considered the possibilities. *Do they need fluids, or do they need pressors?* Two drastically different plans of attack with the same overall goal. As a brand-new nurse, I would have immediately thought *low blood pressure = bolus.* But this time, instinctively, I went straight to the electronic medical record (EMR), scanning for a history of heart failure—because mindlessly pushing fluids could make the situation worse. I checked for jugular vein distention (JVD), listened to lung sounds, and assessed overall fluid status. The answer wasn't more fluids; they needed vasopressors to improve perfusion.

For the first time, I didn't freeze. I wasn't just following orders or reacting—I was anticipating, thinking ahead.

I left work that evening, walking down the long corridor to the staff parking lot. I got in my car, picked up the phone, and called my aunt.

And you're probably thinking, *Umm ... okay? What does that have to do with the story?*

Because after nearly six months of struggling to find my place in the ER, I didn't leave feeling defeated. I didn't go home in tears. I didn't replay the entire twelve-hour shift in my head, overanalyzing every decision I made. I didn't question my interventions with that patient. Instead, I got in my car, picked up the phone, and had a conversation *completely unrelated* to the chaos of the last twelve hours.

And that's when it hit me.

Ah-ha ... This is the feeling.

I wasn't just surviving anymore. I wasn't a scared, timid, uncertain version of myself.

Slowly but surely, I was becoming Nurse Steph—gentle affirmation that I was stepping into the role I had always aspired to. It was finally clicking.

Anyone who enters a new grad residency should expect an adjustment period. It's inevitable. How you decide to navigate that time will make or break you.

When you feel lost—and trust me, you will—it can consume you if you don't find a way to push through. I hear from thousands of new grad nurses around the world, all sharing the same doubts about their choices, their abilities, and their path. The stories you've shared—being belittled, leaving shifts in tears, feeling overwhelmed by the weight of responsibility—echo a common question: *Will it get better?*

Here's what I want you to know:

1. **You are not alone.** I read these messages every day. Every single new grad has felt these same doubts. I felt them too.

2. **Keep pushing forward.** The ability to persevere—despite your own doubts and the doubts of others—says everything about the kind of nurse you are becoming.

There will come a day—and the timing is different for everyone—when things *finally* click. When you'll stop second-guessing every move and realize, *Oh ... this makes sense. I actually know what I'm doing now.*

For me, that shift happened around the six-month mark. Some say it took them a full year. And I know that's a long time to power through—but you *have* to give yourself the grace to get there.

I promise, it will come.

The Follow-Up

One of the hardest parts of being a nurse is lying in bed after a shift, overwhelmed with anxiety—replaying every decision, every action, wondering if you missed something or made a mistake. *Did I chart everything correctly? Did I remember to titrate the drip before I left? Did I overlook a subtle sign of decline? Did I notify the doctor about that critical lab?* No one really prepares you for that—the relentless loop of *what-ifs* that follows you long after you leave the hospital.

But even worse than the doubt is what comes after you *do* make a mistake. Because now, your flaws aren't just your own; they exist in the minds of others, shaping their perception of you and your competence as a nurse. And for some, that weight is crippling.

I'll be the first to admit that I was brutal on myself after my first few mistakes. *Damn, you should have known better. Why did you do that?* The weight of a misstep in nursing feels different than in most other jobs. There's no redo, no do-over—no undo button for someone's literal life.

The first *big* mistake I was a part of had the potential to end my career before it even really began. At the time, I hadn't yet learned all the protocols that would eventually become second nature. I understood the basics but the small, critical details? Those were still taking shape in my mind. For instance, I knew that if a patient presented with chest pain, we needed to capture an EKG within a certain time frame. What I didn't fully grasp yet was what to do with the EKG afterward.

A patient presented to the emergency department with a chief complaint of chest pain. In his mid-fifties, he had left the gym mid-workout because his chest had started to feel, in his words, "full of pressure." With a background in medicine, he knew something wasn't right, so he drove himself to the hospital and walked into the ER to get checked out.

It was a relatively mellow day in the emergency department. On slower days like this, we sometimes take patients directly to an open bed and complete the triage assessment at the bedside rather than in the designated triage room. Why? Honestly, why not? As a new nurse, I appreciated these moments. It gave me a chance to observe the triage process firsthand—the questions asked, the workflow, and how things were done at this particular hospital.

The patient was placed in my colleague's room. Since things were slow, my preceptor and I decided to involve ourselves in the triage process—especially given the nature of the complaint. It was a valuable learning opportunity, a chance to observe and maybe even get my hands in there to help.

The primary nurse began the triage while I stood at the doorway, observing the charting process and watching my colleagues assume their roles. The EMT helped the patient change into a gown, while another nurse placed the EKG leads almost in tandem. The blood pressure cuff was on, vitals cycling within seconds of the patient sitting on the gurney.

From my bird's-eye view, I was lost in my own world of observation—taking it all in—until a voice pulled me back to reality.

"Steph, want to capture the EKG?"

"Sure!" I said as I made my way to the head of the bed. This was something I knew how to do.

"What's your pain level on a scale of 1 to 10?" the primary nurse asked.

"Probably a seven. It feels like a lot of pressure on my chest." He looked slightly clammy.

"I'm just going to lower you down slightly to get this EKG, okay? Hold still—no talking or moving for a few seconds."

"No problem, do what you need to do."

I lowered the head of the bed, and the team subtly adjusted their movements—keeping the momentum going but ensuring nothing interfered with capturing a clean EKG.

"All right, got it."

The monitor screamed STEMI—so obvious it only took a glance. No words were needed. In that silent moment of recognition, the entire team moved as one.

A STEMI (ST-Elevation Myocardial Infarction) is a type of heart attack caused by a complete obstruction in one of the coronary arteries, which supply blood to the heart muscle. This blockage impedes blood flow to the heart, and without immediate intervention, patients are at significant risk for irreversible heart damage or death. Prompt medical intervention is crucial to minimize myocardial damage and improve patient survival rates.

When a patient presents with chest pain, one of the primary concerns is ruling out a STEMI, as it is a time-sensitive, life-threatening condition. Most hospitals have established protocols that mandate the capture of an EKG within a specific time frame from the moment the patient is entered into the triage waiting system. Failure to meet this standard can have serious clinical and legal repercussions. For this reason, chest pain complaints are handled with the utmost urgency.

Patients typically report a sensation of heavy, crushing chest pain, often describing it as if an elephant is sitting on their chest. The pain may radiate to the left arm, neck, or jaw. Additional symptoms can include shortness of breath, nausea, lightheadedness, or diaphoresis (profuse sweating). It is important to note, however, that women may present with more atypical symptoms, such as fatigue, nausea, and discomfort in the back, shoulders, or stomach, making early detection and diagnosis more challenging. This subtle presentation often complicates the identification of STEMI in female patients compared to the more classic symptoms typically seen in males.

As I raised the head of the bed, a colleague nearby said, "I'll print it and get it to the physician." I nodded, trusting that the next critical step was in motion. This was standard protocol—every chest pain patient required an EKG within ten minutes, reviewed and signed off by a physician without delay. This process was essential for identifying life-threatening cardiac dysrhythmias and ensuring high-risk patients were prioritized appropriately.

With that handled, I shifted my focus, scanning the room to see where else I could assist. The team continued working seamlessly, each person absorbed in their respective tasks. A few minutes passed before another colleague spoke up. "Why hasn't the doctor come by yet? Did someone give him the EKG?"

A sudden wave of panic hit me. I turned toward the nurses' station, my mind racing. Had it been printed? Had it been delivered? My eyes darted across the room until they landed on the colleague who had volunteered to print it—now busy in another patient's room.

Oh my God. Did she get sidetracked?

It turned out the patient's EKG never reached the physician. When the doctor finally came by, frustration evident in his voice, he demanded, "Why didn't anyone tell me about this?" That single lapse had thrown off the entire timing of our protocol—and I was the one who had dropped the ball.

The patient was rushed to the cath lab within minutes, where they found a 90 percent occlusion of the left anterior descending (LAD) artery. Thankfully, the delay didn't impact his outcome. But that didn't lighten the weight of what had happened. I couldn't shake the thought that this could have ended so much worse. And I was damn lucky that it didn't.

Still, as much as I wanted to, I couldn't dwell on the *should've, could've, would've.* I was new. I was learning. And after debriefing, I knew that a mistake like this could have easily cost me my job—one misstep away from a very different outcome. While this moment could have defined me as the nurse who failed in a critical moment, I refused to let it. Instead, I had to take it for what it was—an experience that would make me sharper, more aware, and ultimately, a better nurse.

That's the thing about this field—mistakes are inevitable. Some are small, some are serious, but the weight they leave behind is never easy to carry.

You spend every second with your brain running at full capacity, double-checking every medication, following every wacky protocol, recalling every possible adverse effect—and still, mistakes happen. Not because of negligence, not because you don't care, but because you are human.

I also came to understand the deeper art of delegation. In nursing, we are taught that we don't have to carry the weight of every responsibility alone. The profession is, after all, more of a team sport than not. We rely on each other, and we learn to lean on our colleagues to share the load.

However, delegation isn't just about passing off tasks; the true test lies in making sure that what was delegated is *actually* carried out. In fact, the follow-up often holds more weight than the delegation itself, ensuring that the task doesn't just exist in theory but comes to life in practice. Nobody specifically taught me this. And I don't fault anyone for not teaching me this crucial aspect of delegation because, in many ways, it's something you learn through experience. Through moments like this one, when I was reminded in the most profound way that I will never, ever forget to follow up—whether it's asking someone if they've printed the EKG or confirming the physician received it. This is a lesson learned the hard way, but it's one that will stay with me forever.

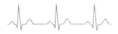

"Don't get too comfortable." Those were my preceptor's infamous words of advice to me as a new grad. And boy, did I come to see the weight of that throughout my residency. For instance, I was working alongside a charge nurse with over a decade of experience in her role—a position that carries far more responsibility and authority than mine. Even she wasn't immune to mistakes. In a moment of checking off her task list, moving on autopilot, she administered eight times the prescribed dose of insulin. Eight times the dose. Let that sink in.

So after everything, my biggest piece of advice when it comes to mistakes is this: Be kind to yourself in the face of your errors, master the art of follow-up on delegated tasks, and never get too comfortable. These experiences were a harsh reminder that mistakes aren't just a rite of passage for new nurses—they can happen at any stage of a career. The key is shifting your mindset from *I'm terrified to make a mistake* to *I'll probably fuck something up at some point, but I'll learn from it and make sure it doesn't happen again.* It's about asking yourself, *What can I do better next time? How can I improve?* That shift in thinking is what separates the inexperienced from the seasoned—the kind of nurse who lets go of perfection and leans into the beauty of being human.

Dealing With Death

I speak from experience here—whether that's a good thing or a bad thing, I'm still not sure. No one *wants* experience with death, but in a way, I'm grateful for mine. It shaped how I deal with it now, both personally and professionally.

When my mom passed away, one of my best friends from high school gave me a journal. A red one—my mom's favorite color. She told me I could write *whatever* I wanted in it. Things I wished I could tell my mom, a recap of my day, checklists—anything. Writing had helped her process her own loss, so she passed the idea on to me.

Over the years, I've made that journal my own. I decorated it with stickers—little reminders that made me smile. "Not Today, Satan," one of my mom's favorite sayings. "Remember why you started," another. Glittery pictures of a brain, tulips, nurse icons—things that make me happy.

At first, I filled its pages with letters to my mom. I wrote about my nursing journey, the day I graduated, how I knew she would have been over the moon to see me get pinned. I wrote about RNExplained and every single detail of its creation. I wrote about the hardest decision I ever made—cutting my dad out of my life—and about the house I bought on my own and the friends I made at my first nursing job. I hoped, somehow, she was still proud of me, still part of it all in some way.

And then, when I started my first nursing job and encountered death, trauma, and the weight of it all, the journal took on a new purpose. It became the place where I unloaded the hardest parts of my job. A space to process the patients I lost, the moments that shook me, the things I couldn't say out loud.

Because dealing with death at work is different. It's not just grief—it's responsibility, detachment, pressure. It's learning how to hold space for someone else's loss while still managing your own.

People always say, "Don't take your work home with you." But of course we do. How could we not? When you pour your compassion, knowledge, and energy into a patient, they don't just disappear from your mind when the shift ends. They linger—in your thoughts, in your heart.

We need somewhere to put those feelings. That's why I started writing down the names of my patients who have died. Not their actual names—nothing that violates HIPAA—but something that reminds me of who they were. "Motorcycle gloves." "Avocado lady." He died with his gloves still on. Her favorite blanket was covered in avocados. You get the idea.

Writing them down is my way of closing my chapter with them. It helps me grieve without letting grief consume me. It's how I honor them, acknowledge them, and still allow myself to keep moving forward.

But one thing I've learned—through loss in my own life and in the lives of my patients—is that there's no right way to grieve. When I ask other nurses how they cope with death, the answers vary. Some work out. Others journal. Some debrief with coworkers or loved ones over a glass of wine. Some meditate. And all of those are valid, powerful outlets.

But the biggest lesson isn't about how you grieve—it's about recognizing that everyone grieves differently. It's about honoring your own process while also respecting the ways others do. Especially in a field where death is as common as the changing seasons.

We owe it to each other, as coworkers, to understand and support each other's grieving habits. Because when we do, something incredible happens: The team becomes stronger, more aligned, and healthier as a whole.

In a minute, I'll tell you a story about when I truly understood this—and the impact it left on me.

Every Rose Has Its Thorn

What happens when the very people you rely on for support and guidance become the ones who tear you down? When an environment, marketed as positive and tight-knit, actually hides an undercurrent of bullying, masked by the facade of teamwork and camaraderie? This is a topic that has weighed heavily on my mind for quite some time, and I've spent considerable thought on how to express it effectively. Workplace bullying and hazing occur in many professions, but in nursing, it's so prevalent that it's earned a notorious saying: "Nurses eat their young."

It was only two hours into one of my first shifts when my manager decided to introduce me to the team. Though I had already made my rounds with my preceptor, meeting new faces, she insisted on doing it again. We approached the nearby physicians' room, and as we entered, she said, "This is Stephanee."

Dr. S, whom I had met earlier in the day, looked up from his chair, a smile spreading across his face. He seemed genuinely happy to see us again.

"Yeah! I know!" he exclaimed. "Did you know she has an entire business educating nurses?" He pulled out his phone, flipping through my social media educational videos.

"Yeah, I know," my manager replied, her tone flat yet deliberate. "She's going to take my job one day."

I didn't look at her, but in my mind, I thought, *Okay, this is the precedent we're setting here?* Was it a casual comment, meant in jest, or was there something more beneath it? Perhaps an indirect insinuation, an offhand remark designed to belittle or undermine. Regardless of intent, I brushed it off, though I couldn't help but feel that I was already marked—already placed outside the circle I had hoped to join.

A few weeks later, I was called into the manager's office with my preceptor, completely blindsided amid our shift. As we approached the door, I turned to her, a sense of unease creeping in. "What's this about?" I whispered, trying to keep my voice steady. She glanced back at me and whispered just as quietly, "I have no idea."

We walked into the small cluttered room, and my eyes immediately landed on my new grad residency director, sitting with a clipboard. The weight of uncertainty hit me like a tidal wave. A knot of anxiety tightened in my stomach. My heart sank, the silence in the room amplified the tension. *What have I done wrong? Is this a random evaluation? Is something about my performance being questioned?* It felt as though the air around me was thick with judgment, but there was no clear reason why.

In that moment, I glanced at my preceptor, my rock during those early months—someone who had been nothing short of a godsend. She was the light I needed to keep pushing forward. Her unwavering kindness and dedication to her patients and colleagues made her the nurse I aspired to be. She was respected by everyone she worked with, always eager to learn and teach—a true embodiment of the nursing profession. And yet now, in this strange and unexpected moment, even her ability to precept me was being questioned.

The conversation was less of a discussion and more of a blunt critique. My manager began listing concerns: how ill-prepared I appeared to the team, how we (my preceptor and I) spent too much time on the computer and not enough in the patient's room. When my preceptor tried to explain that we were using our downtime to learn the EMR, my manager dismissed it as laziness. "You should be doing that in the patient's room, not at the nurses' station," she said.

Then came the real blow: "Charge nurses aren't thrilled to see you on their Saturday schedules."

For context, Saturdays were the busiest days in the ER. It was generally understood that those scheduled on Saturdays were among the strongest nurses, though it wasn't explicitly stated. I had envisioned being one of the chosen for those shifts, so this feedback was particularly stinging.

"Are they going to want you on their Saturdays? Are you going to be the one running to a code? Are you even happy working in the ER? Because, honestly, I can't tell with you."

With each word, I felt the tears welling up, just waiting for one to fall. My heart sank as I realized what was being implied—that I wasn't measuring up, that I wasn't enough. The longer the conversation stretched on, the more it felt like a blade twisting deeper into my chest.

I was in love with emergency medicine. Despite the occasional harsh words from colleagues or the emotional toll of loss, I thrived on the chaos, the adrenaline, the urgency. Every shift was a chance to learn and grow. I showed up with energy and enthusiasm, eager to prove myself. I thought I had built relationships, forged friendships. I believed I was part of something. So why, in that moment, did it feel like I was being pushed farther away?

I tried not to let it shake my confidence, though I have to admit, I left that office in tears. I cried for twenty minutes in an empty patient room, feeling utterly defeated and questioning everything—and everyone—around me. Given the unexpected nature of the meeting and the lack of any formal residency evaluation process, I am convinced that the intention behind it was to leave me feeling beaten. Her words stayed with me for months, and in moments of self-doubt—even now—I can still hear her voice: *Are they going to want you on their Saturdays?* Yet this was only the beginning.

Unfortunately, it was management who was with me when I faced my first patient death. And if you're a nurse, you know how unusual that sentence sounds, but nonetheless, it was my luck that they were present.

Let me tell you—no matter how prestigious your nursing program, nothing truly prepares you for your first death. Sure, they teach you the algorithms, CPR, and to "make sure the bed is at hip level," but there are so many other components to navigate: how to communicate with the family, the role of the scribe, and how to process it afterward—mentally and emotionally. The list goes on. Death is a strange concept to navigate because, depending on the situation, my thoughts on it shift.

Take, for example, when patients arrive *already* deceased, with EMS attempting to resuscitate. In those situations, the worst has *already* happened, and there's no uncertainty about what's coming. We have time to prepare, assign roles, and follow protocol. The pressure, although intense, is predictable.

But when a patient is "circling the drain," it's different. If you're unfamiliar, this phrase refers to a patient who is still alive but rapidly approaching the point of coding, their pulse fading and likely to become absent at any given moment. We do everything we can to stabilize them, but there's always an underlying awareness that the situation is grim. The challenge lies in the constant struggle to change the course, to find that one thing that might make a difference. *What do I need to have ready? Am I mentally prepared for the worst? How soon could this happen? And who can I rely on for support when it does?* The preparation for death is far more daunting than the death itself.

Here's how it unfolded. An older male arrived via ambulance under a Code Alert. In our hospital, a Code Alert indicates that EMS is actively performing CPR during transport, as the patient is in respiratory or cardiac arrest. At the time, I had an available room, so that's where the patient was directed upon arrival.

The roles were filled quickly, which is ideal in these situations, as it allows the team to seamlessly move into position without unnecessary chatter. I volunteered to be the nurse pushing medications, hoping to experience a role different from those I had previously taken during other codes. Next to me was another nurse, managing the second IV for medication pushes and handing me medications from the nurse overseeing the crash cart at the foot of the bed. And who was handing me those medications? My manager.

I know, I know—this probably sounds unusual. A fully staffed day in the ER, and the manager steps into a code role? I had never seen that before either. But nonetheless, when the physician called out a medication, she handed me the ampule, and I administered it.

The patient did not survive.

It was the first time I had lost a patient of my own—and only the second time I had witnessed death firsthand, the first being my own mother. As I learned, the nurse is responsible for an extensive postmortem protocol. So as the code concluded, I collected the necessary paperwork and began the weighty process.

My manager sighed, running a hand over her face. "All right, first things first—time of death. Make sure you chart it exactly as the physician declared."

I nodded, my pen already hovering over the paper. "Okay. Time of death."

She gave a small nod but didn't hesitate before moving on. "Don't forget the postmortem checklist. You need to remove all medical equipment—IVs, catheters, monitors—unless this is going to the medical examiner. If it is, you leave everything in place."

I blinked, trying to process. "Wait, IVs stay in for the medical examiner?"

"Yes. And you must call them to report the death. They'll tell you if they're taking the case or not."

I let out a slow breath. "Okay ... medical examiner first."

"Then you tag the body. Make sure you account for all personal belongings. And if the family is going to take the belongings home, they need to sign for it."

"Toe tag, body bag, belongings ..." I muttered. "Okay."

"You'll also need to make sure the physician completes the death certificate."

I stared at my never-ending list like it was written in another language.

"Oh, and notify the organ donation team," she added. "Even if they're not a donor, you still have to make the call."

"Death certificate, organ donation ..." I repeated.

"Security." She tapped her badge absentmindedly. "If the patient had any valuables locked up, they have to be released to the next of kin. And once they've moved the body to the morgue, call environmental services to clean the room."

I blinked at her, my mind scrambling to keep up. "Right. Time of death, family, IVs out unless the medical examiner takes it, but call the medical examiner first though, tag the body, document everything, call organ donation, fill out the death certificate, notify security, call environmental services." I shook my head, overwhelmed.

She studied me for a beat, then walked out of the room as she said, "That's it."

I stood there for a moment, staring at the paperwork in my hands, feeling the weight of responsibility as I flipped through the forms, trying to remember each step, each procedure.

Two hours passed as I meticulously reviewed every detail, striving to ensure that each task was completed correctly. Around me, the other nurses moved in their usual rhythm, absorbed in their own assignments. As I sat at the nurses' station, finishing up my documentation and discussing the final item on my postmortem checklist with the charge nurse— calling security to transfer the patient to the morgue—my manager interjected.

"Did you get someone to sign for the belongings?" she asked, her eyes scanning my stack of paperwork.

A wave of realization hit me. In the rush of paperwork and the emotional weight of the situation, I had completely forgotten to have the belongings line signed. After spending nearly an hour at the bedside with the patient's son, guiding him through his final moments, it had slipped my mind entirely. I responded, "Shoot, no. I'm sorry. The family member was here, and he took the clothes, but I didn't think to have him sign for them."

"I told you that you needed to get it signed," she replied sharply, her tone edged with frustration.

I apologized, explaining that I hadn't heard her mention it or registered the importance of that detail. My response was calm and steady, not panicked. While I acknowledged my mistake, I'm not the type to make a spectacle of errors; I prefer to find a solution and move forward. Given the intensity of the code and the emotional weight of postmortem care, dwelling on a minor oversight seemed unnecessary. The charge nurse and I resolved the mistake within the hour, and our shift continued.

Unbeknownst to me, however, my reaction hadn't met her expectations. A week later, I was called into her office.

"The way you brushed off the missing signature when I brought it up was completely unacceptable," she said, her voice rigid.

I blinked, caught off guard. It had been over a week since we'd interacted, and I genuinely wasn't sure what she was referring to.

"Your attitude was dismissive and careless, as if it didn't even matter. And then you had the nerve to say you didn't hear me? That's calling me a liar in front of the entire team. It took me this long to confront you because I'm still shocked by how you handled that."

I was taken back. I had never intended to cast doubt on her integrity, nor had I questioned her authority. Yet it seemed she was expecting a different response in the moment—maybe she was looking for me to excessively apologize or show a level of submission that I didn't think was warranted. But that wasn't me, nor would it ever be. Regardless of rank or position, I don't engage in brownnosing behavior. We're all part of the same team.

Her frustration escalated as she claimed that the charge nurse was equally disturbed by how I had handled the situation. The claim unsettled me. *Should I have expressed more emotion?* I don't wear my feelings on my sleeve, and the situation felt—quite frankly—like something to be handled with a level head. But I wondered: *Had I been wrong? Had I mishandled the death in some way?*

I went home that night, reflecting on the situation, feeling terrible about the impact it may have had on my team. The next day, I sent an email to the charge nurse, acknowledging my oversight and assuring her that I had never intended to question anyone's authority or professionalism. The following morning, she approached me with a warm smile and said, "I never thought you handled it poorly."

"Wait, really?" I asked, surprised.

She nodded. "Yes, it was completely fine. I'd honestly forgotten about that issue."

In the end, I could only assume that my manager's reaction was driven by a desire to provoke a certain response from me—perhaps to humiliate me or constantly make me feel less than in this field. And in that, she succeeded. The experience left me questioning my worth nearly every shift. Despite my constant efforts to prove my competence and passion, it seemed like nothing would ever be enough for her. It wasn't just one isolated incident that made me feel inadequate; it was a repeated pattern.

Like the time I asked a colleague to review my charting, hoping for constructive feedback, only to be met with a thinly veiled jab: "You may be successful in life, but this is a whole different ball game, sweetheart."

Or the time, on an unusually empty day with one stable patient, when I noticed a pediatric anaphylaxis was en route. Eager to help, I made my way to the ambulance bay, only for a nurse ahead of me to turn around and say, "Why don't you just stay back here and round on your patients or something? We don't need you."

Or when, while performing a Foley catheter insertion on a confused elderly woman, I asked a medic to help hold her legs steady. As I was trying to find the right spot, he chuckled and said to another coworker, "Man, you're really slow. Do you even know what you're doing?" They both joined in, laughing at me in front of the patient.

Or the time a nurse wrapped her arms around the other new grad and said, "You're my favorite new grad." There were only two of us in the residency program.

For months, I fought to be enough. And it wasn't until years later, after leaving and reflecting on everything I had endured, that I recognized it for what it truly was—classic "eat their young" behavior. I gave more and more of myself, trying to fit into an environment that never truly saw me or valued what I had to offer. Every day, I twisted myself into a version I thought they wanted, constantly striving for approval, for acknowledgment—for anything that might make me feel like I belonged. But the harder I tried, the more invisible I felt.

And throughout it all, I withdrew mentally, observing as the same toxic treatment was directed at others who entered the unit for the first time—students, new grads, travel nurses. It pained me to see the light fade from their eyes, the way they hesitated to ask questions, afraid of ridicule or of what might be said about them behind closed doors. So I made myself a promise: I would never, ever allow anyone else to feel the way I had felt in those early years. No nurse should have to question the worth of what they worked so hard to achieve or exist in an environment designed to make them feel small.

It's ironic to me, witnessing nurse bully culture in full effect. How unhappy must you be in your role to feel the need to tear someone else down? And yes, there is a difference between nurses who

1. lack tact but genuinely aim to provide constructive criticism,
2. are just simply mean bitches.

Yet regardless of intent, both fail to remember that no one ever became a competent nurse without first starting off as a complete disaster. You don't graduate nursing school *as* a nurse—you become one. Over time. Being a nurse is a skill in itself, built upon countless smaller skills we refine every day.

Let me say that again for the people in the back: The job itself—the art of being a nurse as a whole—is something learned, refined, and made your own over time. Give yourself grace. Show up as the best version of yourself. Strive to be the best nurse you can be. Ask the questions. Make the mistakes. And never forget where you came from.

So while I pick up the pieces of the nurse you broke, I hope you find satisfaction in being a contributor to the most toxic work culture known to the profession. After all, every rose has its thorn—and some thorns are harder to avoid than others.

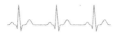

One last thought—regarding the time my manager said I was "too nonchalant" about the code and had a "careless attitude" toward the mistake I made. Her words left me questioning her intent and, for a long while, my own ability to navigate complex emotions in the workplace. I've reflected on this moment countless times, even years before writing this book, always considering what I would want others to take away from it. So here it goes:

The moment my mother died right before my eyes—the moment I changed her into her favorite pajamas and zipped her into a body bag—I became numb. I learned to separate myself from the emotion of death and view it as a task to be done: to change her clothes, to zip the bag, check the box. Done.

Normally, I would preach the importance of not just completing tasks to check a box. I'd say, *Think about what you're doing and why you're doing it.* But when it comes to death, this is how I cope. And the way I handle it is completely okay.

Many people assume that grief should be outwardly visible—crying, showing sadness, or verbalizing emotions. In reality, grief is not linear—people move back and forth between emotions, and some might skip certain feelings entirely. There is no single way to grieve, just as there is no single way to comfort. In nursing, we are taught to follow the Golden Rule: Treat others as you want to be treated. But when a nurse has experienced loss, the Golden Rule isn't enough. Instead, we need to follow Steph's Rule: Be mindful of others' ways of grieving.

My stoic demeanor and calm tone were not *too nonchalant* or *careless*. They were how I process grief. And if my manager had held a debrief with the team after the code, if she had asked about my behavior in that moment—if she had taken a second to see the person behind the situation instead of jumping straight to logistics and criticism—she would have known that.

But I can't meet someone at their low level. So I will, respectfully, hold space for others to grieve in their own way—just as I do for myself.

S + S

If someone were to ask me, *When did you stop feeling like a newbie and step into your confidence?* my mind immediately goes to one specific patient: a two-shift-long interaction that completely changed everything for me.

This was the moment that shifted my mentality from *I'm just a new grad nurse* to *Oh no, honey—I am that nurse.*

Five years later, I still replay every emotion from that experience: frustration, disbelief, anger, pride, accomplishment, betrayal, and even moments of feeling completely lost. It was the best and worst story of my career, but it was also the day that changed my entire professional demeanor.

So when people ask me that question, I dance around the story. I share what I felt and what I learned about confidence at a surface level. But I've never actually told anyone the details— because the emotions behind it are something that took me *years* to debrief. It's the one memory of finding my confidence that I *should* feel the proudest of. I *should* be able to answer that question with excitement, ready to share a damn good story. Yet it remains the hardest to talk about.

This is the most raw, real story of the internal battle in a new grad nurse's mind. It was the moment I found my voice.

And I'm ready to talk about it.

I had just started my shift, and the night was still dark. The ER had a steady flow of patients and EMS runs—nothing out of the ordinary. Around 2200, EMS called in a patient from home. Let's look at the triage note:

2200:

32-year-old female, AOx4, NKDA. Chief complaint: mild sob. Was receiving infusion of Remicade at home with home health nurse when the nurse stopped infusion early d/t sob complaint. Satting 99% on RA at home and in triage. Otherwise well-appearing. Able to speak in clear sentences without impairment. VSS. Denies chest pain, nausea, vomiting, or diarrhea. Hx Crohn's disease. Pt's second time receiving infusion at home, denies complaints or complications prior. Denies any other complaints at this time.

Her medical history noted Crohn's disease, and she was receiving Remicade (infliximab) infusions through a home health nurse. Crohn's disease is a chronic inflammatory bowel disease that can affect any part of the digestive tract, from the mouth to the anus. It is characterized by persistent inflammation that damages the intestinal walls, leading to flare-ups and a range of symptoms. The key immune cells involved include macrophages,

T-helper cells, dendritic cells, and neutrophils, which release TNF-α and other pro-inflammatory cytokines. This triggers a cascade of immune responses, increasing vascular permeability, damaging the mucosal barrier, and leading to chronic inflammation, ulceration, and fibrosis.

One treatment option for moderate to severe Crohn's disease is Remicade (infliximab), a TNF inhibitor classified as a biologic disease-modifying antirheumatic drug (DMARD) and a monoclonal antibody. Given what we know about Crohn's disease and the class of this medication, we can say that Remicade will stop (inhibit) the *normal function* of TNF-α, a key driver of the harmful immune response. In professional terms, it specifically targets and neutralizes TNF-α, reducing inflammation and preventing further immune cell activation in the gut.

Due to frequent flare-ups, her primary care physician had prescribed at-home Remicade infusions, administered by a home health nurse every eight weeks over a two-and-a-half-hour infusion period. The first infusion she'd received eight weeks earlier had no complications. However, during the second infusion, the nurse stopped the infusion early due to the patient's mild complaints of shortness of breath and requested further evaluation before continuing treatment. When the patient arrived, she described the sensation as barely noticeable—so faint that she almost regretted mentioning it in the first place. Over and over, she reassured us that she felt completely fine. And after assessing her, every health care professional involved in her care—including myself—agreed with her.

We connected her to the monitor, applied the EKG leads, and took her vital signs, which were stable and consistently within normal range. In typical ER fashion (and precaution), we started 1L NS KVO via 20G in the right antecubital (AC) and took some basic labs. As she alternated phone calls between her husband and primary doctor, she kept repeating, "This is so stupid. I need to go home. Why am I here?" For a moment, we all exchanged looks, wondering, *Why* is *she here?* She appeared walkie-talkie and healthy, and even the ER physician agreed that she seemed fine. However, he suggested we monitor her for a couple of hours before discharging her, just to be safe.

For me as her primary nurse, that meant keeping her on the continuous monitor and validating her vitals ... and that's about it. While I tended to my other three patients, I checked in with her periodically to assess her status and ensure there were no changes from her baseline. And that's exactly what I did.

Let's take a moment to discuss the role of the home health nurse because you'll soon find out she's the real hero of this entire story. When a patient receives an infusion of any kind, it is the nurse's responsibility to consistently assess for potential complications. These can range from something as subtle as erythema at the infusion site or a 1 percent change in oxygen saturation. It can include a facial grimace or even the most obvious signs of a severe reaction, such as a sudden drop in vital signs or a direct "I don't feel okay" comment.

On top of being detectives, nurses are expected to know the specific signs to watch for when administering certain medications. Take vancomycin, for instance? Red man syndrome—slow down the infusion. Blood products? Watch for shortness of breath—stop the infusion immediately. Potassium? If the patient complains of burning, we assess the site and dilute or slow down the rate. You get the idea. It's our job to be vigilant, to know the warning signs, recognize any subtle changes, and take action.

For patients receiving Remicade, the side effects can include chest pain, fever, chills, itching, and trouble breathing, with the infamous worst-case scenario being escalation to anaphylaxis. A pretty standard set of potential side effects but ones that always need to be in the back of a nurse's mind. With this knowledge, the home health nurse made the decision to stop the infusion early, despite the patient's complaint being incredibly minimal. It was almost a comment made under her breath—something the average person would probably ignore. But the nurse noticed it. She wanted to be cautious, and though it might annoy the patient, that inconvenience could be what ultimately saves their life.

That's the reality in health care: There's no one-size-fits-all presentation. Some people may appear outwardly fine, but their internal homeostasis is drastically off, and we can't always see that with the naked eye. Other times, they truly are as fine as they seem, and you're simply grateful that being extra cautious was all it took. Patient presentations can vary by gender, nationality, and even personal pain tolerance too. Cultural differences can also influence how symptoms are expressed or reported. Again, all things we consider in our mental checklist. But when we say *monitor*, it's not because we want to waste your time—it's a precautionary measure. We choose to monitor, check your labs, and observe you because we understand that no two cases are alike. The *what-ifs* are always there, and we're doing everything we can to prevent anything from going wrong.

At that point, it had been about an hour since I last checked in with my patient. I had done rounds every fifteen minutes to make sure she didn't need anything, and there had been no changes in her vital signs. She was still on the phone with her primary doctor, expressing how she wanted to go home and how this whole thing felt like a waste of her time. I went into the room to take another blood pressure reading, and as I did, I overheard her physician on the phone reassuring her that nothing was wrong and that she'd likely be discharged soon. Her doctor agreed that it was just "dumb protocol" and encouraged her to distract herself during the long wait.

After finishing up, I stepped out to check on my other patients, returning about thirty minutes later for another quick "Hey, I didn't forget about you. Just popping in to say hello." But this time, she was off the phone and mentioned that her chest "felt funny," and she experienced that slight shortness of breath again. She described it as a brief episode that lasted just a few seconds and quickly passed.

As I processed her complaint, my first instinct was to check her vital signs. If a patient mentions shortness of breath, my training tells me to check their oxygen saturation—it's the *first* thing we do. Her pulse oximeter was reading 98 percent on the monitor, and she appeared clear to auscultation. All other vital signs were within normal limits.

But then I reminded myself: *We treat the patient, not the monitor.* So despite the normal readings, I reported her symptoms to the doctor. He reassured me that we should continue monitoring, as there were no critical changes in lab results or vitals to suggest immediate intervention. Fair enough.

Fifteen minutes later, I returned to her room and asked how she was feeling. This time, she told me that the shortness of breath had returned. I glanced up at the screen and saw that her oxygen saturation had dropped to 95 percent. I checked the sensor on her finger—it was still intact, and this was her true reading.

At that point, I was confused. A thought ran through my mind: *Huh, okay, this is a change, but not necessarily a huge one, yet it's still a change.* She still appeared okay otherwise, and her labs were stable. But I couldn't ignore the fact that something was different. Going through my mental checklist, I considered my next steps. What could I do at this moment? I grabbed a nasal cannula and set the oxygen to two liters, thinking this might help provide her some relief. I updated the doctor again, and he suggested we admit her overnight for further monitoring.

I went back into her room to explain the plan to her— that we wanted to admit her just to be extra cautious and that she would eventually be moved to a room upstairs once one became available. It would be quieter upstairs, she could get some rest, and hopefully, she'd be feeling well enough to go home in the morning. Even though we were making this decision based on her self-report and vitals, she was clearly frustrated. It was obvious she didn't want to be there. She wanted to go home to her husband and two young children, and you could feel the tension in her voice as she expressed how unnecessary it all felt. As the nurse, I understood her frustration and recognized that it wasn't personal to me. So I continued my care, left the room, and carried on with the night.

Some logistic background: Once a patient is admitted from the emergency department, their care transitions from the ER physician to the attending physician. Even if the patient hasn't physically moved to an inpatient bed yet, they are no longer under the ER physician's supervision. This means that, as the ER nurse, I now have to contact the attending physician for any questions or concerns—unlike in the ER, where providers are just steps away from the nurses' station for quick, face-to-face discussions.

You see where I'm going with this? ER nursing operates on a completely different dynamic when it comes to physician-nurse communication and response time. One of the perks of the ER is that the fast-paced environment forces a high level of collaboration, with the entire interdisciplinary team quite literally within arm's reach. But once a patient is admitted, I essentially shift into "floor nurse" mode for their care—while still juggling my other three ER patients—until I can hand off the patient to a nurse upstairs.

Her status had officially changed to "admitted," but she was still waiting for a bed. Under normal circumstances, this wouldn't be a huge deal; a bed would open up in a reasonable amount of time. Sure, it's a bit of an adjustment for an ER nurse used to fast, direct communication, but it was manageable. However, these weren't normal times. These were pandemic times. Entire hospital floors had been converted into COVID wards, admissions for observation were at an all-time high, and bed, staff, and resource availability were at an all-time low. Instead of a quick handoff within the hour, we were holding admitted patients in the ER for ten to fifteen hours—sometimes more than twenty-four.

As usual, I went in to check on her and assess whether the nasal cannula had improved her condition. But with just a quick glance, something felt off. She looked worse.

My assessment instincts kicked in immediately—her breathing seemed different. Earlier, she had been chatting away on the phone, but now she was taking slightly bigger, more deliberate breaths, sitting taller in bed—an instinctive maneuver the body uses to maximize oxygen intake. My eyes gazed at the monitor. Heart rate: 104, slightly tachycardic. Oxygen saturation: 93 percent, dropping again.

"How are you feeling?" I asked, already knowing the answer but using it as another assessment tool—gauging not just her words, but her effort in speaking.

"I can't seem to catch my breath," she said, motioning toward her chest as she attempted to take a deep breath.

I immediately called over a colleague—because when in doubt, *always* get a second pair of eyes. Mind you, by this time,

I was officially on my own as a new graduate nurse. I had a solid grip on critical thinking and carrying out interventions, but like I always say, this job is never a one-person show. We work collaboratively for the sake of our patient's well-being, and if I need to brainstorm potential solutions to a problem I'm having, you know damn well I'll be doing it with *everyone*— nurses, techs, charge nurses, physicians, even security if it comes down to it. We ALL have valuable insight, and in moments like these, that collective knowledge can make all the difference.

We stood at her bedside, mentally running through our checklists. *What can we do right now to help? What needs to happen next? And what are the worst-case scenarios if this keeps going south?*

I bumped her oxygen up to six liters, hoping for some improvement, and sent a message to the admitting physician with my findings. Based on past experience with attendings who weren't physically in the department, I decided I'd give him five minutes to respond before I called him directly.

In the meantime, I had three other patients to tend to.

One was a sweet elderly man who had taken a ground-level fall at his senior home. He needed to be evaluated for a potential hip fracture, as his clinical presentation showed shortening of the right leg. His X-rays had already been done; now we were waiting for radiology to read them and determine the next steps.

Another was a young woman with suprapubic abdominal pain for the past three days, radiating up her right flank. I had already run her urine sample and sent it off for culture and sensitivity. In the meantime, she was waiting for an ultrasound to rule out the "potentials"—pregnancy, appendicitis, pelvic masses or lesions, renal calculi, etc. Since this was well into the night, resources were limited, and ultrasound techs weren't readily available. She understood the delay and was okay with it, but I knew the waiting game wasn't ideal.

Another was a middle-aged man with complaints of intermittent palpitations that had started three hours ago. He said they began after dinner with his wife and kids, with no clear triggers or cardiac history. His pupils were dilated, he was tachycardic on the monitor, and he startled easily whenever I walked into the room. With my experience so far, I'd have bet on some kind of stimulant—cocaine, maybe? You'd be surprised how many seemingly composed, well-put-together people have ended up in the ER due to drug use. Then again, we don't put it past anyone. Just to cover all bases, I hooked him up to the monitor, phlebotomy drew his cardiac labs, I started IV fluids, and we collected a urine sample for drug screening.

Five minutes passed—still no response from the attending on my patient with shortness of breath. So I called. He answered in a quiet tone, probably winding down for the night. I laid it out in typical Situation, Background, Assessment, Recommendation (SBAR) fashion: *32-year-old healthy female, received Remicade at home, stopped by infusion nurse due to shortness of breath, NKDA, worsening respiratory distress, 93% O$_2$ on 6L NC,*

visibly increased work of breathing. I had tried a nasal cannula, bumped
her to 6L, but her oxygen saturation kept dropping.

"I think you should lay eyes on her so we can come up
with a plan together," I suggested.

"Bump her to 10L. I'll come down at some point," he
replied.

Max her out on a nasal cannula and wait? That call left me
uneasy—not because I doubted him, but because I felt like
more could be done, and *I* was the one watching her every
movement. Maybe I should have suggested something specific
in my SBAR, but truthfully, I didn't know *what* that something
was. I had exhausted what I knew—sit her up, apply oxygen,
increase said oxygen, gather opinions from coworkers and the
charge nurse. Now, I was just supposed to wait and watch?

But I was a new grad, still learning the fine line between
advocacy and overstepping. Not wanting to be dramatic, not
wanting to challenge hierarchy, I did exactly that. I waited. And
I watched.

Her husband called just after midnight, asking for an
update on his wife's status and whether she had been moved
upstairs yet. I explained that we were still waiting for a bed,
but with how slow things move overnight, it was likely she'd
be staying in the ER for the night. I assured him I'd keep her
comfortable down here until a bed became available.

"She's having some trouble breathing again, so I gave
her extra oxygen to help her feel better. The doctor will come

down soon to check on her. For now, we're keeping a close eye on her, and I'll keep you posted if anything changes," I said.

He seemed reassured and thanked me for keeping him updated.

Thirty minutes passed and still no sign of the attending. Despite the late hour, the ER was alive with movement—every room full, every nurse working in parallel, managing their own patients and tasks. My confusion shifted to nervousness as she showed no improvement on 10L NC. Now, 90 percent O_2. Trusting my nursing judgment, I escalated her oxygen support, switching her to a non-rebreather. I sent another message to the attending. Again, no response.

Minutes stretched into what felt like hours as I stood in the doorway with my charge nurse and resource nurse, my mind racing in a million directions. Part of me was extremely nervous—thinking about what could happen next. *Are we missing something? Is this my fault? What if she codes?*

At the same time, I was rifling through the file cabinets in my brain, grasping for anything—any intervention within my scope that could buy us time, turn this around. Overwhelmed didn't even begin to cover it. I had three other patients, but right now? *None of them existed.* Fuck everything else—I was not leaving her side.

And then there was the part of me that felt utterly lost. Because no matter how hard I tried, no matter what I did, my hands were ultimately tied—waiting for a physician who wasn't there.

Two minutes. That's all it took—standing in that doorway—for her oxygen saturation to plummet into the 80s. 86 percent, to be exact.

In my five years as a nurse, I had never, not once, stood at the foot of a patient's bed and watched them deteriorate so rapidly.

Agitation set in—a telltale sign that oxygen was slipping away from her brain. Her eyes darted around the room, confusion taking hold as she forgot where she was. She clawed at her IV lines, tore the mask from her face, gasping between broken sentences. Then she was on her knees in the middle of the bed, tripod position, hallucinating birds and butterflies in the room. 84 percent oxygen saturation.

"Where are my kids?" she muttered repeatedly.

My coworker and I held her firmly, keeping her from pulling out her lines as I shouted for someone—anyone—to call a rapid response, to get help into the room. We tried our best to reorient her.

"You are in the hospital" I said. "We're going to take care of you."

But were we really taking care of her? Was this the best we could do? I was doing everything I had been taught—following the chain of command, trusting the judgment of those with far more experience than me. I was trying to be the best nurse I could be. And yet, none of it was making a difference.

It was the most surreal, helpless, and frustrating moment I had ever experienced. And in those two minutes, something in me shifted. A switch flipped.

I will never, ever forget that feeling. I was watching this woman slip away before my eyes, holding her struggling body, and I'd be damned if she coded in front of me. The fear of stepping on toes, of being "too dramatic," of respecting the hierarchy of the interdisciplinary team—gone. None of it mattered.

I didn't care what anyone thought of me or my nursing expertise. She was *my* patient. I may have been a new grad, but *I* knew what was best for her. She needed to be intubated, and it was going to happen—immediately.

A glance down the ER halls and I see the attending physician, strolling down like he was casually window shopping. I was livid. *How dare he take his sweet time after dozens of phone calls and messages? How dare he walk those halls so nonchalantly while we're here listening to her slip in and out of hallucinations, begging not to die?*

We met in the doorway of his patient's room.

"How's it going?"

How's it going? It's a fucking shit show, and where the fuck have you been? I screamed internally.

I cut straight to the chase. "I have no idea what's going on with her but her sats are eighty-three percent and dropping. She needs to be intubated now."

He glanced briefly into the room. "Oh yeah, looks like she needs that. Let's prep the supplies." *Well, no shit, Sherlock.* Then without urgency, he walked to the physician's desk, sat down, and waited for us to prepare the room.

In the meantime, every available nurse and tech jumped in to assist with gathering the necessary supplies, retrieving restraints, and preparing the room. The respiratory therapist (RT) was on his way. Given the patient's decline and the impending intubation, the nurse-patient ratio was adjusted to one-to-one. While we focused on the intubation, the charge nurse reassigned patients as needed.

Sixty seconds passed in preparation. 80 percent oxygen saturation.

I approached the physician, who was sitting at a desk, casually flipping through his cellphone. "We're ready to intubate," I informed him.

He grabbed a stack of sticky notes and a pen, turned to me, and wrote "S + S" on the sticky note, encircling our initials with a heart. He peeled it off and handed it to me.

"Why didn't you call me sooner? I would've loved to hear your voice sooner," he said.

For a split second, the hospital around me fell silent. The beeping monitors, the distant chatter, the overhead pages—everything faded. I stood there, stunned, unable to muster a response. It felt as if the blood had drained from my head. All I could think was the sheer disrespect—toward me, yes, but more so toward my patient. Without a word, I turned and walked toward the room, preparing for the intubation.

"Am I going to die?" she gasped between breaths. "Please, don't let me die. Where are my kids?"

As the etomidate was administered, I guided her gently to supine, lowering the head of the bed and locking eyes with her. Her hand gripped mine in terror, her words broken with hallucinations, her voice pleading, "Please, don't let me die."

"We're going to do everything we can, I promise," I said, my voice firm but gentle. "We're going to help you breathe now."

Shortly after 0100, she was successfully intubated.

For the next six hours, she remained my sole focus until the day nurse took over. But even after leaving the hospital, I couldn't shake the thought of her decline. I went home, yet she never left my mind. And when I returned for my next shift, she was still there—still holding in the ER, waiting for an ICU bed. I asked the charge nurse if I could take her assignment again. After everything, I needed to see this through—not just for her, but for myself.

When people ask me *So when did you stop feeling like a newbie and step into your confidence, Steph?* It started with her. A battle against self-doubt, against the hierarchy, against the fear of looking incompetent, and locking eyes with someone pleading, "Don't let me die."

As a new graduate nurse, fresh on my own and without a preceptor, I was drowning in self-doubt. *Am I doing this right? Am I missing something? Do I look stupid? Am I overstepping?*

They say, "Don't be afraid to ask questions." But when I do, I'm met with smirks and condescending sighs.

They say, "Never hesitate to ask for help." But when I do, I'm met with eye rolls and rushed explanations.

They say, "If you're unsure, get a second opinion." But when I do, I'm met with a backhanded compliment about lacking confidence.

So tell me: What the fuck is a new grad *supposed* to feel? Because it is *so. damn. hard.* to be new.

It is *so damn hard* to silence the whispers behind your back, to keep moving forward when you feel like you're drowning in judgment or self-doubt. It is *so damn hard* to stand your ground when the very people you look up to make you feel small.

But then, there was her.

Her oxygen was dropping, her body was failing, and in that moment, *I* was the only one standing between her and the worst-case scenario. I *had* to step into my confidence. I exuded confidence I didn't yet feel, demanded respect for my knowledge and skill, and trusted my gut—because *she* needed me to.

That's how I found my confidence. Through advocacy. Through learning, in the most visceral way possible, that nothing— nothing—matters more than speaking up for your patient. Not fear. Not hierarchy. Not ego.

And I know it's easier said than done, trust me. But little by little, shift by shift, whether it's catching a wrong medication dose, getting a smooth IV insertion on a screaming baby the first try, or offering a suggestion that a doctor takes seriously— these moments slowly build your confidence. And don't get me wrong, a little twinge of self-doubt will keep you diligent too! But be patient with yourself. Over time, that confidence *will* overpower the doubt.

As for my patient—she lived. A late-onset transfusion reaction. Extremely rare, with an incidence of only 1–3 percent. I'd like to think that it was my advocacy that saved her life. But if I'm being honest, I give credit to the home health nurse who trusted her gut.

I spent two days with her in the emergency department, titrating her drips and meticulously watching her labs. Her husband decorated the room with family photos. I found myself staring at them often, listening to stories about her kids and their family vacations.

Two days later, a bed finally opened up in the ICU. She was transferred, and after that, I never heard from them again.

As for the sticky note ... I still have no words for that.

One Curtain Over

"Shut the fuck up!" the teenager in handcuffs screamed as I tried to convince him to provide a urine sample. "I'm not doing it. Get away from me!"

He'd come in around 1700 during that lull period in between day and night shift, led by a police officer we had seen one too many times before in this ER. Upon initial assessment, the patient appeared physically well— AOx4, his clothes appropriate to weather, skin color appropriate to ethnicity, clean, and in no acute distress aside from the fact that he appeared in our ER and chose violence today. I noted minor abrasions grazing the bilateral hands and arms, but the patient was otherwise well appearing. He sat on the gurney, angry and yelling, refusing to provide a urine sample, while the police officer stood by with a look that screamed, *Just another Sunday night.*

In the room next door was a middle-aged man who'd arrived via EMS as a Code Alert—a dad who'd been standing outside an Italian restaurant, waiting to pick up a take-out order for his family, when a street racer lost control and plowed into the restaurant, striking him. It was a heartbreaking moment—a reminder that life can change in an instant.

The room was a whirlwind of activity, everyone working seamlessly to save the victim. Nurses and EMTs pressed against his chest in steady, rhythmic CPR, their faces taut with focus, while others prepped medications. To the trauma-trained eye, the outcome was painfully clear—he was already gone. Blood pooled on the floor, forming sticky trails beneath the footsteps of staff moving fluidly around the code. Our team had perfected the art of organized chaos, so much so that you might never guess a horrific situation was unfolding just one curtain away. That's where I was—one curtain over—still trying to coax my patient into providing a urine sample. The MD stood firm, determined to test for intoxication. But with no cooperation from the patient, we pivoted to a serum tox screen instead.

The TV in the corner of the room was tuned to the evening news, broadcasting a report about the accident in front of the Italian restaurant. Caught in a moment of shared stillness, my coworkers not involved in the code and I paused at the nurses' station to watch. On the screen, a blurry clip showed the driver being handcuffed by LAPD. My head turned in confusion as I glanced to my right—at my patient. Turning back to the TV, the next image showed the mangled facade of the Italian restaurant. I looked again to my right. This time, one curtain over.

One man had his ribs cracking under deep compressions, a team battling to save his life. The other, just feet away, cursing about going home and demanding his handcuffs be removed. My patient had not a care in the world except his own record— no idea he'd killed anyone. And especially no idea that the person he'd killed was one curtain over. None of us did. The connection between the two didn't become clear until the news report played on the TV overhead. Up until then, we were just doing our jobs—treating them as two separate stories.

I continued to do just that—my job—after learning this information. Yes, my patient was a murderer. And yes, it was my job to take care of him. There's an unsettling duality in being a health care worker. The patient in front of me, regardless of their actions outside the walls of the hospital, still needed care. As I worked, I found myself wrestling with this internal conflict—my mind recognizing the severity of his actions while simultaneously thinking, *Damn, this young kid has an entirely different life path now, and he has no idea. I feel bad in a way.*

I didn't know him. I didn't know if he had siblings, if he was close with his parents, or if he had dreams of becoming something more than the man who'd ended up in my care. I didn't know if he'd ever been to the beach, if he was someone who'd ever seen a sunset and paused to appreciate it. I didn't know if he'd gotten into street racing with the wrong crowd or if his parents ever scolded him for speeding before. What I did know was that, in that moment, his life was no longer his own; it had shifted in a way that none of us could reverse.

But none of that matters to my role as a nurse. I'm not here to piece together someone's story or judge them based on a snippet of their life I happen to see.

The ethics of care don't come with a moral clause. Our job is to provide care, to help this person in front of me—no context required.

It's a strange and humbling concept to care for someone with no understanding of what led them here, but it also highlights the beauty of the ER. A melting pot of people come through our doors, each carrying their own unique story. We don't usually get much context about who people are or what they've done (unless they're a foundation member—then management just loves pointing them out). Shit, what we really get is a fifteen-second recall of your age, allergies, last bowel movement, and whether or not you have chest pain. We know 0.0001 percent about you when we step into your room—and yet we care for you regardless. Without context. Our focus is on what you need, not what you've done wrong.

The general lack of context actually helps us stay unbiased and focused on our jobs—but even when we have more context, we still deliver the same level of care. I often get asked, "Why do you like the ER so much?" I'll say it once, and I'll say it forever: the vulnerability.

Emergency departments see some of the most vulnerable populations—people who have found themselves unable to care for their illness, their child, their mother, etc. Others end up in the ED after a moment they never thought they'd endure: a traumatic car accident, a heart attack, an overdose, their first seizure, etc.

An incarcerated male being medically cleared for prison.

A young woman asking for a pregnancy test, worried her boyfriend will find out she cheated on him.

A teenage kid who was told to eat staples and die by his classmates, and so he tried it.

All situations where a person has found themselves in a vulnerable state and needing *my help* to make it through. The opportunity to look at a patient as more than just their circumstances. To take my ever-growing knowledge and critically apply it to *save a literal human* ... That's why I love the ER so much. Because everyone deserves to be treated with dignity, even when life has thrown them into the most chaotic and vulnerable (and sometimes illegal) moments.

If you're reading this with no medical background or with minimal knowledge and thinking *Steph, you lost me at Code Alert*, this theory extends far beyond the health care field. I adopt this mentality in all aspects of my life—to care without context. We often don't know the battles people are fighting just one curtain over.

Split and Run

Night shift. 0200.

I typically hesitate to use the "Q word" in the ER (aka "quiet") because it's practically a curse that guarantees all hell breaking loose. In this case, even though I would describe the evening as dark and mellow to carefully avoid the superstitious Q word, all hell broke loose anyway.

It all started when my coworker had gone out to the front of the hospital for a smoke break. The world outside was eerily still—dead silent. Not a soul lingered except for the distant silhouette of the valet man, barely visible at the end of the hospital entrance. To the average person, the night brings stillness. But to the health care worker on night shift, the hospital hums with its own energy—a quiet yet relentless buzz that reminds us the work never truly sleeps. I'd often joke with my coworkers, "When the rest of the world sleeps, we witness some of the most larger-than-life medical emergencies." And how beautiful it is, in a way, that the rest of the world doesn't have to see the things we do when the sun sets. They remain blissfully unaware of the tragedies unfolding, a naivety that is probably for the best. It's an experience that's nearly impossible to explain unless you've worked a night shift yourself.

After spending roughly two years working some variation of nights, I've gained immense respect and admiration for the staff who make it through those hours. Traumatic emergencies with limited resources, no management to call for backup, makeshift solutions when supplies run low—it's a world like no other. You lean on your colleagues in a way that forges an unshakable bond, relying on one another to make it through the chaos. I'd like to think my *figure it out* attitude was shaped in those years, in that unique world where resourcefulness and teamwork became instinct.

Much of the general public doesn't know about what we call a "homie drop-off"—a grim scenario when someone drops off a dead or dying person outside the hospital entrance and speeds off. In most cases, the driver doesn't want to get in trouble or was involved in something illegal. That's what happened with this patient—one I'll call Jane Doe.

A fancy sports car pulled up beside my coworker, mid-drag. The driver gestured to get a wheelchair for the person in the passenger seat. My coworker stubbed out his cigarette, grabbed a wheelchair, and worked with the driver to get the person seated. While he was focused on assessing the patient for immediate issues, the driver took off. If no one had been out there, it's likely he would have abandoned the person at the entrance or in the ambulance bay behind the hospital, which happens all too often.

After the driver sped off, my coworker was left with a limp, unconscious body in the wheelchair. As a nurse, that's when your critical thinking kicks into high gear: *What could be wrong with this patient?* You sort through a massive internal checklist within seconds—one that forms from a combination of training and experience. Everyone's list tends to be a little bit different, but we hit the high points and run a quick process of elimination.

Do they have a pulse? If not, we need to start CPR. Is this an overdose? It could be alcohol or possibly drugs. Are they bleeding from anywhere? Is this a gunshot wound victim? Do I see a stab wound? Do we suspect any sort of abuse, such as signs of choking, bruising, or neglect? What's their physical presentation? Does it appear they are dirty, possibly unhoused? Do they have good hygiene? How old are they?

In this case, the patient had no ID and couldn't communicate. Our first rule-out on the mental checklist: pulse.

Absent.

Without hesitation, my coworker rushed her inside, his movements swift and purposeful. "Call a code," he told the front desk staff, his voice steady despite the urgency.

While he worked quickly, the rest of us were still in the ER, casually going about our tasks, completely unaware of the emergency unfolding just beyond the doors. Then the overhead speaker crackled to life.

"Code Blue, main lobby, hospital."

The message was as clear as it was chilling—someone was dead.

In that instant, the weight of the words sank in. "Code Blue, main lobby, hospital" we heard again. The sound of the announcement echoed through the walls, and the confusion among us was almost tangible. The room seemed to freeze for a moment.

And yes, I know what you're thinking: *Get up and help!* It was literally a two-second moment of confusion, okay? In those few seconds, the gears in my brain were spinning, trying to make sense of it. Code Blues didn't happen in the lobby, of all places. They were typically seen in the ER, ICU, or sometimes even MedSurg, but never the main lobby.

I stepped into the hallway, hoping to see what was happening. The polished vinyl flooring stretched out before me like a never-ending tunnel, filled with the distant sounds of shoes scuffing against the surface and soft murmurs of voices.

Then out of the corner of my eye, I saw him. My coworker came running down the hall, pushing Jane in a wheelchair. The scene felt like it was unfolding in slow motion—her body limp, nearly sliding off the chair. Her head lolled to the side, eyes closed, and there was no sign of life. Sweat glistened on my coworker's forehead as he struggled to catch his breath, his panic barely contained.

"CPR. We need to do CPR," he said urgently, barely able to get the words out between heavy breaths.

Jane was a woman who otherwise looked healthy, except for the fact that she was unconscious and had no pulse. We got her to a bed, started CPR, and administered Narcan; our second rule-out on the mental checklist: overdose.

> Narcan (naloxone) is an opioid antagonist, designed to rapidly reverse the effects of opioids by blocking their receptors in the brain. If an overdose was the cause of her condition, Narcan would typically restore breathing and consciousness within minutes. If no response occurs within two minutes, a second dose is typically administered.

When the Narcan didn't work, we moved on, continuing to methodically run through the checklist.

As a new graduate in the ER, I was taught to focus on three things: lines, labs, and EKG. These were the pillars of nursing intervention, the first steps in unraveling any chief complaint mystery.

I remember sitting at the nurses' station with my colleagues during lulls, absorbing their wisdom like scripture. They would ask, "What's the first thing you do when you walk into a patient's room?" The answer was always the same: lines, labs, EKG. Over time, the pattern became instinct. Of course, this rule didn't apply to the man with a stubbed toe or the child with something stuck in their ear. But you slowly learn that *most* complaints warrant the trio. A general rule of thumb: If the complaint is from the abdomen up, get the trio. (Remember, though, medicine is fluid, and the rules bend to the patient in front of you.)

We start lines to establish IV access, ensuring we have a route for fluids, medications, or emergency drugs like epinephrine. In emergency medicine, there's an old saying: "Two is one, and one is none." A single IV site is never sufficient in a crisis. That's like knowingly setting yourself up for disaster when abdominal pain turns out to be a sudden aortic dissection or when you're pushing insulin during a hyperkalemia protocol. If one line fails, you'd better have a backup.

We draw labs because our mental checklist demands we consider every possible cause. Labs are more than just numbers on a screen—they are a window into the patient's body, revealing what they cannot say. Is the patient's blood sugar dangerously low? Are they anemic? Do they have a lethal electrolyte imbalance? We check arterial blood gases for oxygenation and acid-base status, cardiac biomarkers to rule out a heart attack, and a comprehensive metabolic panel to expose any hidden abnormalities.

Finally, we capture an EKG to assess the heart's rhythm. In this case, there was none. No electrical activity. No pulse. So we resumed compressions.

Our mental checklist guided us through each protocol, each possibility. We ruled out hemorrhage—no gunshot wounds, no signs of trauma. We pushed medications, we pumped her chest, we cycled through every maneuver designed to pull a person back from the abyss.

But sometimes, despite everything, it's just too late.

She was already gone.

As she lay lifeless on the gurney, we had a moment to truly observe *her*—as a human not just a body. In the chaos of emergency care, our focus is always on the immediate, the critical, the logical. We move with purpose, driven by training, instincts, and urgency. But once the crisis has passed and the adrenaline subsides, we're left to face the reality of who that person was.

At first glance, she appeared young. Her face, smooth and unmarked, still carried traces of the life she'd lived—freshly manicured nails and tattoos splashed across her legs. But as we began postmortem care, her arms told a different story. Track marks, faint but unmistakable, ran along her skin, a quiet testament to the struggles that had shaped her.

The person who dropped her off didn't just leave *her*, they threw a duffel bag out of the car before speeding away. The bag, frayed at the edges and covered in scuff marks, was retrieved by a security guard from the lobby shortly after we called her time of death. And when the police arrived, they confiscated the bag as evidence. Inside, the clothes were unwashed, wrinkled, and hastily stuffed into a disheveled pile. The fabric carried a stale, unpleasant odor, the kind that clung to it despite the passing hours. Beneath the clothes, wedged tightly between them, was a journal—its leather cover cracked and worn from years of use. The pages inside were a chaotic mess, some torn out, others folded or frayed at the edges. Handwritten scrawls filled nearly every page, the ink smudged in places as though written in a hurry or in desperation. One entry, in particular, stood out—a raw confession about longing to reunite with her children yet burdened with the pain of not having custody.

It's hard not to wonder about the life our patients lived before they arrived. Just like my street-racing patient who crashed into the Italian restaurant, we rarely know the full story. I try my best not to take the little information I have and spiral down rabbit holes of *How did you end up here?* Stopping myself from thinking this way keeps me detached from the situation, which is what we *want* as a nurse. To get attached means losing the ability to be objective, to think clearly, to "do the right thing," even when sometimes doing the right thing means allowing someone to die.

In Jane's case, it was reasonable to conclude she had overdosed long before she was dropped off—tragically, the Narcan hadn't been enough to bring her back in time.

Jane's case—though it didn't end the way we had hoped—reinforced the power of mental checklists. In fact, no one really talks about how important it is to build them. It's like an unspoken piece of homework when you're a new grad, but this isn't the kind of homework with a due date—it's never-ending. It's something that can't really be taught, because it's your own personal way of critical thinking.

Every situation you encounter, every adverse reaction you witness, and every mistake—yours or a coworker's—adds to your checklist. It's a This could go terribly sideways or I already messed up once I'm not doing that again kind of mentality that sharpens your ability to anticipate and respond.

I like to think of them as file cabinets in your brain. When a patient complains of chest pain, you instinctively pull open the cardiac and abdominal drawers, running through possible diagnoses, questions to ask, potential complications, medications, and anticipated interventions. If a patient shows up with aphasia and confusion, you unlock the neurologic drawer and start digging. You get the idea. The beauty of this system is that no two people have the exact same checklist. Collectively, our unique experiences help fill in the gaps during emergencies—the "potentials," the "what-ifs," and the "we-should-try-this's."

Don't get me wrong—it's definitely not as easy as it looks. This is where new grad nurses struggle the most, and I can speak from personal experience when I say the learning curve is steep. It's not just about memorizing the right interventions; it's about developing the mental agility to open the right file cabinets and instantly visualize all the possibilities—like a conspiracy map with pins and strings connecting symptoms, causes, and interventions. The sheer volume of information you have to process in a single moment can be overwhelming, and no textbook can truly prepare you for that.

I have two points to make about this:

First, the transition from textbook knowledge to real-world application is incredibly difficult, and you are not alone in that struggle. Too often, I see new graduate nurses being overly critical of themselves for freezing during a code or struggling to think critically under pressure. If you're in that place right now, don't give up on yourself. *This is normal.* Your brain is building those file cabinets—one by one. Honor your own pace as you navigate this learning curve. You are doing the best you can, and that is more than enough.

Second, never forget how remarkable it is to possess the skills of a nurse. No one outside of health care will ever fully grasp the speed at which we process these mental checklists— in mere seconds. No one will truly understand how lifesaving it is that our minds work this way. And as you face more situations, your instincts will sharpen, your confidence will grow, and your ability to respond will become second nature. So if you're struggling, remember this: *You are in the process of becoming extraordinary. Trust yourself and recognize that you're crafting a mind that most people would strive a lifetime to develop. It doesn't happen overnight.*

"If They Die, They Die"

I started traveling a year and a half after becoming a nurse, for a few reasons. The most superficial? The money. Let's be real—it's a huge factor in the decision to travel as a nurse. The pay is simply better—don't ask me how or why, it just is. In some cases, it's nearly double what staff nurses make hourly.

The second reason? Freedom. As a traveler, you're not tied down to a single hospital. If you don't like the environment, the management, or anything else, you're not stuck. Most contracts last only a few months, giving you the flexibility to extend or move on. That kind of freedom is unmatched.

And then, of course, there's the travel itself. You get to work in places you'd probably want to visit anyway. As a young nurse with nothing keeping me in one place, this was one of the biggest perks. My mindset was simple: I could always become a staff nurse again when I wanted to settle down, but for now, travel nursing offered the perfect blend of adventure and professional growth.

I get asked this question all the time: "When did you know you were ready to travel nurse?" or "How long should

I be a nurse before traveling?" The truth? There's no one-size-fits-all answer. Everyone's journey is different, and that's the beauty of this profession—you decide when you feel ready. But I know that's not the answer you were hoping for, so here's my general rule of thumb based on personal experience.

If you started your career in a new grad residency program (like I did), finish it. Most residency programs last about a year, and you *need* that time to truly settle into your role as a nurse. I could go on an entire tangent about why residency programs are invaluable, but we'll save that for another chapter.

In general, I recommend new nurses complete at least one full year before even considering travel nursing. That being said, I've had friends who jumped into travel nursing right at the one-year mark, and while it may sound intimidating, it's more common than you'd think! Personally, I waited until I had a year and a half of experience before making the switch. By then, I felt confident in my skills, had learned everything I could from my hospital, trusted my critical thinking, and was ready to challenge myself further. But that was *my* timeline—yours might look different. Maybe you'll want two years under your belt or even three. That's totally fine!

One important thing to keep in mind: Most hospitals require at least two years of experience to qualify for a travel position. Some accept nurses with just one year (which is the type of hospital I chose), but those positions are sparse. This requirement exists because you're expected to jump in with little to no learning curve. Most travelers get one day of orientation (if that) and maybe a single shadow shift before being thrown into a unit where the staff has been working together for years. You're expected to function at the level of an experienced nurse, with minimal preparation.

So with all of that being said—choose travel nursing when *you* are ready. Anyway, back to the story.

I chose to travel to a hospital in an underserved community—one where patients truly needed health care the most. I wasn't interested in working with a patient population that was solely entitled and demanding. Instead, this population is often living with the harsh realities of poverty. Their vulnerability is layered: the fear of not being seen, of being ignored, of feeling invisible in a system that doesn't always meet their needs.

It's my role to advocate for them, to stretch the limited resources we have, and to provide care that, in many cases, is better than anything they've received before. And what's incredible is how grateful they are for it. The opportunity to be their first step toward recovery, to bridge that knowledge gap, and to advocate for their care is exactly what *this* population needed.

Beyond serving an underserved population, hospitals in these areas are often underresourced, requiring nurses to adapt and make do every shift. And call me crazy, but I actually *like* that challenge.

There's something about working in a hospital that doesn't have all the bells and whistles. It pushes you to think critically in a different way, to ask yourself, *What can I do with what I have? How can I improvise to make this work?* It forces creativity, adaptability, and problem-solving on a whole new level.

And then there's the teamwork. As a day shift traveler, that stripped-down, resource-limited environment reminded me of my night shift days. The same sense of camaraderie, the same *make it work* mentality. In underresourced settings, that tight-knit bond naturally forms—because you have to rely on one another. You lean on each other, problem-solve together, and get through the trenches as a team. That kind of bond is rare.

My first week as a travel nurse at this hospital, I had a six-hour orientation. I followed a nurse around to see what the unit was like, where everything was located, and the important extensions I'd need. That was it. The very next shift, I was on my own, thrown right in like I had been there for years. I walked into the break room that morning, knowing no one, and thinking to myself, *Ahhh, I feel so new and alone right now.* The nurses looked at me—some smiled, some kept to themselves with their AirPods in. I don't blame them though; it was the crack of dawn, and I wouldn't be very social either.

The charge nurse came in and started her morning huddle, talking about the hospital's poor stats on medication scanning, how the nurses need to stay on top of ensuring all meds are scanned into the Medication Administration Record (MAR). I was shocked by this conversation. I'd come from a hospital that was incredibly strict about scanning medications—down to the minute it was pulled from the Pyxis and scanned into the MAR. So neurotic that there were times we'd have to come in on our day off to fix our scanning or documentation just to meet the hospital's standards. Going from that environment to one where the scanning rate was so low that they had to huddle about doing better was eye-opening. That should've been my first red flag.

My patient ratio was one to four, which I was used to. The huddle ended, and we went out to find our assignments. Being new to the facility, I didn't know anyone's name. While everyone casually walked up to their night shift nurse without a second thought, I was trying to find "Nurse Waldo" in a crowd of people at shift change.

That's one caveat to travel nursing—you're in a constant state of being lost. Just as you begin to familiarize yourself with the layout, the phone extensions, and the names of your colleagues, your contract ends, and you're right back to square one in a new environment. It requires thick skin and the courage to ask questions without fear of looking clueless. Because I can promise you this: You'll be asking *hundreds* of questions, and you'll need to embrace that vulnerability without hesitation.

I located my night shift nurse and received report on three patients she was handing off. To my relief, the exchange went smoothly. Though I was navigating an entirely new EMR system and had no instinctive knowledge of where to find supplies in an emergency, I was slowly finding my footing. I introduced myself to my patients as their day nurse, then spent any spare moments familiarizing myself with the unit—poking through cabinets, exploring the med room, and stocking my rooms how I'd always known them to be. That small sense of familiarity brought me calm in a state of feeling lost.

By midday, all my morning patients had either been discharged or transferred upstairs. I couldn't help but compare the different protocols and ways of doing things to what I once knew. But honestly, that's the challenge of travel nursing—letting go of habit and routine to embrace change and adapt to a new way of doing things. It challenges you to combine the methods you're accustomed to with fresh approaches you learn elsewhere—sometimes realizing there's a better way than what you were taught.

At that point, I had three new patients. A six-month-old infant had rolled off the bed while the mother was in the shower. Since it was an unwitnessed fall, she was understandably worried, and her instincts were spot-on. Although the baby showed little to no immediate signs of concern, a CT scan revealed a subdural hemorrhage. As soon as the results came back, I started the transfer process to a higher-level pediatric hospital.

A woman in her mid-fifties with bilateral wrist pain after falling while gardening. She denied hitting her head or losing consciousness but had limited range of motion in both wrists. X-rays confirmed bilateral wrist fractures, so she needed double splints, an ortho consult, and help with virtually anything involving her hands.

Then there was a middle-aged man, brought in by ambulance from the airport for intoxication. Airport staff had called 911 as precaution, and EMS transported him here to sober up. I started an IV, gave him some fluids, and moved on with the rest of my tasks.

It was noon, and the department was overwhelmed, flooded with patients in varying degrees of health—severe respiratory failure needing intubation, chest pain workups, and blood transfusions. The sheer volume of high-acuity cases made it clear that the unit was running on the bare minimum—short-staffed, stretched thin, yet somehow still pushing forward. They called it their norm. I could see it in the way the nurses moved, their exhaustion hidden behind well-worn routines, their bodies running on autopilot. Wanting to be as useful as possible, I jumped in where I could—helping the new grad nurses with their hard IV sticks and grabbing medications for nurses who were consistently playing catch-up.

"Steph, you're going to take the patient coming in EMS, eta two minutes." Let's look at the triage note:

1232:

56-year-old male, AOx4, NKDA. Chief complaint: right-sided weakness x3 hours. LNW: 0900. Patient reports being on a morning walk with his wife when he first noticed weakness in his right arm, describing it as "too weak to carry the dog leash." He didn't think much of it until he got home and experienced the same sensation in his right leg. Denies gait disturbances. Right hand grip strength: 3/5, left hand grip strength: 5/5. Patient denies tingling in both upper and lower extremities. No aphasia or dysarthria noted on exam. Otherwise well-appearing. Able to speak in clear sentences without impairment. Denies chest pain, nausea, vomiting, or diarrhea. Denies any other complaints at this time.

In triage:
HR: 98
BP: 183/88
O₂: 99% RA
RR: 18
BG: 134 @1232
NIHSS: 7 @1233

The signs of stroke in this patient are textbook, but there's a complexity to the critical thinking required—let's peel back each layer. At the heart of this diagnosis is the ability to quickly recognize stroke-like symptoms. A stroke occurs without regard for time. While it's easy to spot stroke symptoms when a patient first presents in the ER, we must remember that they can also develop while a patient is hospitalized for an unrelated issue. That is why, regardless of the type of nurse you are, it's crucial to remain vigilant in recognizing and assessing these symptoms throughout the duration of admission. We've all been taught the B.E. F.A.S.T mnemonic, a useful tool for recalling the key signs of a stroke. I strongly encourage anyone reading this to become well-acquainted with it:

B – Balance: Sudden loss of balance or coordination

E – Eyes: Sudden trouble seeing in one or both eyes

F – Face: Facial drooping or uneven smile on one side of the face

A – Arms: Weakness or numbness in one arm. Ask the patient to raise both arms—does one drift downward?

S – Speech: Slurred or difficulty speaking. Ask the patient to repeat a simple sentence

T – Time: Time is brain! If any of these symptoms are present, call for help immediately

Next layer: the differentials—what other medical conditions could this be, aside from a possible stroke? In other words, what conditions mimic the presentation of a stroke? This is a critical consideration, which is why certain tests are included in a Code Stroke workup—to specifically rule out other potential causes and ensure we're on the right path toward the correct treatment. The *biggest* similarity to be cognizant of? Potential hypoglycemia. A stroke and hypoglycemia can mimic each other, as both conditions can cause sudden neurological symptoms such as confusion, weakness on one side of the body, difficulty speaking, and altered consciousness. Essentially, both conditions disrupt normal brain function due to inadequate blood supply, whether from a blockage in the case of a stroke or low blood sugar in the case of hypoglycemia. Without proper medical evaluation, it can be difficult to differentiate between the two. So next time you hear the physician ask, *What's their blood sugar?* now you understand why. This is the layer of ruling out differentials.

The final layer? Timing. With stroke, "time is brain." You've probably heard that phrase before in your studies or throughout the hospital, but what does it *really* mean? Simply put, the sooner we intervene, the better the chances of preserving brain tissue and minimizing long-term deficits. *This* is where the true urgency lies in stroke care—and why we must move quickly through those first two layers of critical thinking to reach this final layer.

If you remember anything during a Code Stroke, let it be this: Get the last known well time (LNW). *When was the last time anyone saw this patient at their baseline?* This single piece of information determines eligibility for life-saving interventions like thrombolytics or mechanical thrombectomy. Without it, treatment options become limited, and every passing minute means more irreversible damage.

Most hospitals approach Code Strokes in a similar way, but since I was new to this hospital, I wanted to clarify their specific protocol.

"Hey, what's your stroke protocol?" I asked a group of nurses gathered at the nurses' station as EMS wheeled the patient in on a gurney.

Typically, a resource nurse accompanies the patient to CT, and once they return, the patient is handed off to the assigned nurse based on staffing and patient ratios. Sometimes, the resource nurse keeps the patient; other times, the primary nurse upon arrival takes over, with their other patients being redistributed.

Ideally, a suspected stroke is a one-to-one assignment, as the nurse must perform neurological checks every fifteen minutes until CT results are back and a treatment plan is determined. However, in real-world nursing, staffing shortages often make strict one-to-one assignments in the ER unrealistic. In these cases, a nurse may have a two-to-one assignment, balancing stroke care with a lower-acuity patient.

Regardless, this is how I've always known it to be—the safest approach for both the stroke patient and the rest of the assignment while also making the best of the resources available.

They stared at me, as if I had just asked a question from another planet—one they'd never heard before. It was a look that reminded me of something out of *Mean Girls*, cold and uninviting, completely devoid of compassion or empathy.

"Do I go with the patient to CT while someone takes my other three patients? Or do you have a stroke team? Is there a specific person who goes with the patient?"

One nurse responded, "*You* go with the patient," and the others seemed to nod in silent agreement, as if that answer had settled the matter.

"Okay, no worries, that's fine with me! So who's going to watch my other three patients?" I asked politely, genuinely curious.

Another nurse chimed in, "Nobody."

Nobody? I stared blankly for a split second, processing the response. Surely she wasn't serious, but the look on her face said otherwise.

"If they die, they die." She shrugged, as if this was just the way things were done around here.

If they die, they die. Let that sink in.

Anger and confusion hit me—the sheer nonchalance in her voice, the way she let those words slip through her teeth as if they meant nothing. *If they die, they die.* It wasn't just what she said; it was *how* she said it. Cold. Emotionless. Completely vacant of the empathy that should be at the core of nursing.

Not on my watch, I thought.

I couldn't help but imagine the roles reversed. What if she were the one lying in that hospital bed, frightened, vulnerable, hoping that the people trained to care for her actually cared? How would she feel if, in that moment, the response she got was *If you die, you die?* It was unthinkable. I questioned her character. Her purpose. How she had gotten this far in a career built on compassion. And yet the silence from the other nurses around her told me she wasn't alone in this mindset. No one corrected her. No one pushed back. That muted agreement was almost as loud as her words.

And then I zoomed out. Maybe this wasn't her. Maybe this was what the system had turned her into. Maybe she *wanted* to care but this was the result of years of burnout, of being stretched too thin, of constantly being forced to choose between patients because there simply weren't enough hands to go around. Or maybe she lacked a positive management system that provided her the space to do this job happily. And while that might explain it, it didn't excuse it. Because no matter how broken the system was, or how shitty they had set up her environment to work in, I couldn't wrap my head around a nurse—someone who had once chosen this path to help others—losing sight of what that truly meant.

I looked at her and said, "Absolutely not. That's not happening. Someone needs to watch my other three patients."

Sure, I was new to this ER and didn't know how they ran things. But I knew what was right. I didn't care what they thought of me. I pushed back against the charge nurse, and eventually, she found someone to cover my other patients while I took him to CT.

It was determined that he had suffered an ischemic stroke, requiring the timely administration of alteplase—a powerful fibrinolytic—within a critical therapeutic window. That kind of situation is *why* we have policies and standards of care. It's *why* we can't let desensitization or burnout dictate how we treat people.

I didn't need to work at this hospital for years to see that there were major flaws. But if we're being honest, *every* hospital has its flaws. It's a give-and-take career—what are you willing to put up with in order to do this job? I chalk up that nurse's behavior to her becoming jaded. She'd been worn down by the poor environmental conditions, the constant fight-or-flight mentality, the immense pressure to save lives with inadequate resources, and the need for support when more people call out than show up.

I never want to become like her, but I know it's all too common. There's a certain level of jadedness that comes with being a nurse, and I don't think you can avoid it entirely—or even that you should. I always say, "Walk a mile in our shoes and see if you don't end up with a little bit of a jaded edge yourself." You try seeing one of the worst child abuse cases you can think of, see them not knowing how to react because that trauma is the only stability they know, and try not to get jaded when the next patient repeatedly pushes their call bell because they "need" ice in their water.

This job is heavy. It can make you hard if you let it. However, there is a fine line between being jaded and losing your compassion.

A certain level of emotional response—whether it's frustration, sadness, or jadedness—is a natural part of caring for others in such intense situations. It's an inevitable consequence of bearing witness to so much pain, and it's part of how we process that weight. But if you can endure all of that without becoming just a little jaded, then you probably don't care about your patients at all.

As the outsider travel nurse, there was an expectation for me to fall in line with how things were done. Within reason, that makes sense—but not when it comes at the expense of patient safety or humanity. Hearing, "If they die, they die," felt like yet another "initiation," much like what I'd experienced with the man who had maggots or the time I fought with the attending to lay eyes on my transfusion reaction lady. Once again, I found myself in a mental battle, questioning whether I should stand my ground. But this time, I was much more comfortable advocating for what was right. I had learned that fitting in couldn't come at the cost of my core values as a nurse.

It's natural, especially as a new grad, to want to fit in, to overextend yourself, and to fall into the trap of people-pleasing while proving yourself. But eventually, you reach a point where you find your voice. You stop caring so much about others' opinions. You come to realize that doing what's right for your patients is far more important than being accepted or fitting into a toxic norm. You learn when to have your teammates' backs and accept their support, but more importantly, you know when to stand firm for yourself and the people in your care.

Because at the end of the day, would you ever want to look in the mirror and say, *They died because I let them?* If you can live with that, maybe you've lost something essential to being a nurse. But for me, I'll continue to stand up, speak out, and do everything I can to protect my patients—even if I'm the only one who will.

The "Right Way"

"Chart like you're going to court" is a phrase every nurse hears, but it takes on a whole new significance when you find yourself on the witness stand.

I learned that the hard way when, three years after a routine shift, I was called to testify in a lawsuit against the hospital. *Three years.* In that time, I had cared for hundreds—maybe thousands—of patients. There was no way I could recall the specifics of that encounter on my own. My only safeguard? The nursing notes I had written in the chart.

In this case, my documentation wasn't just a record—it was a shield. A patient had physically assaulted a fellow nurse, and *my* charting was the key evidence that protected him from false accusations. That experience solidified a lesson I'll never forget.

Charting isn't just about meeting a requirement or checking the boxes—it's about protecting yourself, your patients, and your colleagues. Because when memory fades, the documentation remains.

And here's the irony: The very thing that safeguards your license—the one thing that protects everything you've worked so hard to achieve—gets barely a mention in nursing school. One of, if not *the*, most critical aspects of the job is glossed over in our education. Instead, we're expected to learn it on the fly, in real time, while caring for actual patients. As if learning how to save lives wasn't enough, we're also supposed to figure out how to protect *ourselves* at the same time. The paradox is striking—and, frankly, problematic. But I digress.

Newly hired nurses typically receive about two weeks of orientation before working on the floor with a preceptor, sometimes three weeks for specialty units like the ER or ICU. During this orientation, you're introduced to the essentials of being a new grad nurse as well as the specifics of your unit—whether it's interpreting EKGs, managing ventilators or tracheostomies, or handling OR supplies. You're also given a brief overview of the hospital's charting system—emphasis on *brief*, since it's usually limited to just one to two days.

One or two *days*.

A fleeting glance at a system that holds the power to protect—or jeopardize—our entire license.

In my experience, the only exposure to documentation before this was during clinical rotations in nursing school, when we sat next to a nurse as they charted. And when I say *as they charted*, I mean we were more spectators than participants. We observed what the nurse was actively working on in real time, but the deeper nuances of the process were often lost on us. Luckily, once you become the nurse and are on the floor with your preceptor, that's when the *real* learning begins: how to navigate flow sheets, what to chart, what to leave out, and the documentation protocols for different codes.

Here's the catch though: Despite the immense importance of accurate documentation, there's no formal curriculum or structured training to teach us the "right way" to document. Honestly, has anyone ever learned the "right way?" Instead, we rely on our preceptors—who, like us, learned through a mix of experience and trial and error. It's a system based more on word of mouth than on official guidelines. And while I'm deeply grateful for the guidance my preceptor provided, the reality is that we're all essentially learning from a game of telephone, where best practices are passed down informally, with little oversight or consistency. It's unsettling to think that, for something so critical to our license, there's no formalized approach—just a patchwork of practices passed on by those who, unfortunately, fell victim to the same unstructured system.

Once you've oriented yourself to a charting system, documentation tends to be *relatively* consistent across different systems. I say *relatively* because each hospital has its own specific requirements based on compliance standards and how they prefer to cover their bases. For example, when charting for a stroke, the core elements will generally be the same—such as documenting the LKW time, National Institutes of Health

Stroke Scale (NIHSS) score, and completing the hospital's version of a Code Stroke flow sheet. However, some details may differ from hospital to hospital—like documenting the time the patient left and returned from CT, specifying which stroke screening tools were used, assessment time frames, or noting the time the neuro MD was at the bedside. See where I'm headed with this? While the core aspects of documentation may seem straightforward, it's the nuances—the small details and hospital-specific requirements—that can make all the difference in the accuracy and legal integrity of your charting.

I charted for a patient who wasn't under my care, and three years later, a lawyer contacted me to testify on the case. Yes, I know that sounds a bit bizarre, but let me set the scene.

It was a Monday—a day infamous in health care for being one of the busiest of the week. Apparently, no one wants to work on Mondays, so they head straight to the ER for a doctor's note to excuse them. Sneaky, sneaky! And of course, it was right at shift change, the time when the ER is at its most frenetic. Double the staff, double the noise, as day shift hands off reports to night shift. The air crackles with exhaustion and fresh evening faces, the ER buzzing with the pace of *Let me give report so I can go home.*

We'd just wrapped up our morning huddle when I made my way to the nurses' station to check the whiteboard and see which nurse I'd be taking report from. The hallway was a maze of gurneys, each room packed to capacity, and sixty-three patients waiting impatiently in the lobby.

As I walked down the hall, I couldn't help but notice a young man on a gurney, shouting obscenities at no one in particular, his words hanging in the air like a toxic cloud. Unrestrained. Clearly, the day shift nurses had long since tuned him out, their faces impassive, utterly unfazed by his tirade.

"What's the deal with him?" I asked the nurse sitting at the computer near his bed.

"Well, he's completely wasted, so we're just letting him sleep it off," she replied, barely glancing up. "Came in with his mom—she's in Bed 13A, intubated. Apparently, she fell down the stairs? Brain bleed."

I raised an eyebrow, skepticism written across my face. The patient in question was still bellowing in his bed, unaware of anyone or anything around him—a man in a world of his own.

I continued toward the whiteboard, scanning for the nurse assigned to my beds. As I reviewed the assignments, I noticed a male nurse was assigned to the loud patient in the hallway. A small wave of relief washed over me. If you're a woman in health care, you understand why.

Half an hour passed, and I was easing into my routine— checking the supply stock in each room, signing off on the crash carts. I had finished getting report from day shift, gathered my to-do list, and made my rounds introducing myself to each of my patients. The ER was still a chaotic symphony of noise— no signs of slowing down anytime soon.

I was on my way to run a urine sample when I passed the still-yelling patient in the gurney. Just as I did, I caught his night shift nurse introducing himself.

"Hey buddy, my name is John. I'll be your nurse tonight. Let's keep things smooth in the hallway, all right?"

That didn't sit well with him. His voice, already slurred with intoxication, rose into a furious snarl.

"Remember who the fuck you're talking to, bitch. Where's my mom? You fucking bitches are keeping me away from her!"

I ignored the outburst and stepped into the utility room to run my urine sample, closing the door behind me. The muffled hum of the ER continued outside, but for a few blissful seconds, I enjoyed the rare, short-lived silence.

A minute later, I pushed open the door, printout in hand, ready to move on with my shift. But as I glanced left, I saw him. The patient was now on his knees in the gurney, still spewing profanity at John, his rage barely contained.

"Listen, we're not going to talk like that, sir. I'm not doing this with you," John said, his tone calm but firm.

And then, in a split second, the patient lunged—fists clenched, ready to swing.

I was trapped.

The patient's gurney blocked my path on one side, the heavy utility room door on the other. The only way out was through him.

Beyond the chaos unfolding in front of me, the ER carried on as usual—staff hustling through the halls, immersed in their own tasks, oblivious to what was happening. Maybe they were just used to the sound of raised voices, so no one thought twice about it. Maybe it was because shift change had everyone locked into their own to-do lists. Either way, I was the only one to bear witness.

The patient threw a flurry of punches at John. John reacted on instinct, shoving him back onto the gurney to protect himself. A second of eerie stillness followed—just long enough for me to process what I'd just seen.

Technically, we're not supposed to touch patients like that. We're supposed to let them lunge, punch, hit, bite, scratch—whatever they throw at us—without fighting back. But what was John supposed to do? Just stand there and take it?

I stood frozen, still gripping my patient's urine results, my mind racing as I realized I was cornered. I couldn't grab security, couldn't slip past without walking straight into the altercation.

So I did the only thing I could. I yelled.

"Code Gray!"

The words barely left my mouth before someone—thankfully—hit the emergency button. A second later, the ER snapped out of its collective daze. Nurses and security rushed in, the small encounter quickly escalating into a six- or seven-person brawl as they fought to restrain the patient.

In the end, they got him restrained—wrists secured to either side of the gurney. He stayed there and was fine, eventually.

John, on the other hand ... Well, I wasn't so sure.

As the only witness to the incident, I understood that my documentation would be critical for any future discussions. At the time, I assumed it would be reviewed by the charge nurse or management—a routine witness account of what had transpired. What I didn't anticipate was just how significant my charting would become years later.

Recognizing the gravity of the situation, I knew my documentation had to be meticulous. It was essential to establish that my coworker had been attacked without provocation and to ensure there was a clear, unbiased record of events. While he documented his own account, an independent witness statement would provide crucial support. Because if there's one thing I've learned about nursing, it's that we always have each other's backs—looking out for one another extends *far beyond* patient care.

I carefully recorded a detailed, objective account of the altercation, outlining each action, reaction, and verbal exchange. My goal was to create an indisputable record—one that accurately reflected what I saw, what the security footage would confirm, and what truly happened in that moment. Months went by, and I heard nothing more about the situation, assuming it had been handled internally and resolved without further issue.

Three years later, I had moved on to a different hospital—caring for countless patients in the interim, the incident long forgotten. In truth, I had encountered many more instances of combative behavior toward nurses, and this one had faded into the background like so many others.

Then, unexpectedly, I received a call from a lawyer representing John. The patient had filed a lawsuit against both him and the hospital, alleging violence. As the legal team prepared their case, they combed through the medical records—and there it was: my documentation, providing a clear, unbiased account of the incident. A picture vividly painted by *my* words.

It was a lesson I wouldn't fully grasp until years later: You never know who will revisit your charts or just how much weight your words will carry.

Think of charting as painting a clear picture of exactly what happened in that moment. Anyone—whether they work in health care or not—should be able to read a patient's chart and visualize the situation with absolute clarity, without needing additional context. <u>That</u> is how you should chart.

I don't care if someone says, *We're told to only chart by exception,* or *Our system uses flow sheets instead,* or *Nobody reads the nursing notes.* That's bullshit. Chart your observations. Chart direct quotes from the patient. Document who you received report from or who gave you a critical lab result—with exact names. Chart the time a patient left for diagnostics and when they returned.

I would much rather be the nurse who charted in full detail than the one who left gaps—only to be called years later with nothing to reference while standing on a witness stand. Some might argue, *Extensive nursing notes leave room for interpretation by lawyers and auditors.* And they may be right! But the former is just as true too. And yet, this is just another round of the game of telephone we play in health care—because who's really going to tell us the "right way?"

In my eyes, the right way is to chart thoroughly and with intention—be direct, be factual. If you see it differently, then by all means, do it your way. Just remember: The moment you assign yourself to a patient, your name is permanently attached to their record. You are now a witness to whatever unfolds. Be mindful of that responsibility.

Since this experience, the gravity of proper documentation has stayed with me. So I turned to some of my legal nursing colleagues—the ones who review nurse documentation firsthand, dissecting it in courtrooms and legal proceedings. Keep in mind, this isn't legal advice, nor am I practicing law. Rather, this is a collection of nursing expertise as it applies to legal matters. There aren't enough pages in this book to cover all the dos and don'ts of nursing documentation—but I'll leave you with some of our favorites:

#1 Be mindful of backcharting. Backcharting is completely acceptable—and let's be clear, patient care *always* comes before documentation. *People before paper.* Best practice is real-time charting, but in the middle of a code, it's simply not feasible. Your priority is hands-on care.

That said, backtiming your charting comes with a caveat: Be mindful of your time stamps. You can't be in two places at once. If your documentation shows that you checked restraints on two different patients at 0800 in separate rooms, you've just created a legal red flag. Accuracy matters—not just for liability but for the integrity of patient care.

#2 "Will continue to monitor." Those four words make defense lawyers cringe and plaintiff attorneys cheer. Why? Because too often, nurses who write them document a patient's decline without *actually intervening.* The problem isn't just the phrase itself—it's what it represents. You are documenting what you *will* do, which gives a false promise to the intervention. It gives the illusion of attentive care while masking a failure to recognize and act on *gradual* changes in a patient's condition.

Take this case: One evening, I received a report on an intubated overdose patient. She was young, covered with a gown and blanket while the ventilator handled her breathing. During my initial assessment, I noticed her abdomen was slightly distended, giving me the illusion that she was pregnant or developing ascites. This hadn't been noted the day before, and her urine test was negative. After the nurse finished giving report, I asked, "Is she pregnant too?"

She blinked. "Pregnant? What?"

Despite charting every hour, she had completely missed the subtle, *progressive* changes in the patient's abdomen. By the end of her shift, the patient's bladder had swollen to nearly two liters—dangerously close to rupturing.

And that's the problem with "Will continue to monitor." It's a placeholder, not a plan. Writing those words without taking action—without notifying the physician, reassessing the patient, or documenting follow-ups—turns a nurse into a legal target. And often, rightfully so.

So what should you write instead?

Try: "See interactive flow sheets for assessment and care," or "No further issues noted at this time." If the patient's condition remains stable, "Assessment unchanged."

These phrases confirm that an assessment was performed and demonstrate critical thinking. They show that you actively evaluated whether the patient's condition had changed since the last nursing note. If it *had* changed, your documentation should clearly reflect what was different, whom you notified, and what actions you took.

#3 If you didn't document it, it didn't happen. Blank spaces on a chart aren't just oversights—they're vulnerabilities.

When documentation is incomplete, it creates dangerous ambiguity. Was the blank space left because the treatment wasn't given or because the nurse forgot to chart it? A patient who claims they didn't receive care has a much stronger case if there's no documentation to prove otherwise—even if you administered the treatment, there's no way to verify it without a record. These blank spots can also lead to clinical consequences: missed interventions, repeated procedures, delayed care, and serious safety events. So how do you fix it? Use *N/A* when something doesn't apply. Clearly note refusals. And never assume someone else will chart it. Your documentation protects your patient—and it protects you too.

Don't Get Too Comfortable

If emergency nursing is a high-speed roller coaster, the psychiatric side is the part where the track suddenly disappears. The rules are different, the risks are higher, and the stakes? They shift by the second. One moment, you're having a calm conversation, and the next, you're dodging a handful of feces or sprinting to hit the Code Gray button. (Yes, the feces was really thrown at me.)

Caring for psychiatric patients in the emergency department demands a level of vigilance unlike anything else. You have to be sharp—fully aware of your surroundings and meticulous in your documentation—because every single assessment and nursing note matters. It's not just about their vitals; it's about their words, their behavior, the smallest shifts in body language that could mean the difference between a peaceful shift and full-blown chaos. And if you think you've seen it all? You haven't.

"Don't get too comfortable," I warned my nursing student as we walked the halls of the emergency department.

"The second you let your guard down, they'll find a way to manipulate you—verbally or physically."

Psychiatric patients play by different rules, and as nurses, we have to adapt. Over time, I've learned what works, what doesn't, what keeps you safe, and what will leave you blindsided. Before I tell you this story, let me give you a breakdown of what it really takes to be prepared for a psychiatric patient in the ER—because understanding the magnitude of it is just as important as the story itself.

Psychiatric patients are *supposed* to be an automatic one-to-one monitoring with a sitter. That's the policy, at least—but as I've mentioned throughout this book, real-world nursing rarely follows the textbook. In the Emergency Severity Index (ESI) triage system, psychiatric patients are classified as Level 2. Typically, we associate ESI Level 2 with conditions that pose a *potential* threat to life, limb, sight, or organ function if not treated quickly—stressors like active chest pain, altered mental status, or an inability to manage one's own secretions. But this level *also* includes psychological distress: suicidal ideation (SI), homicidal ideation (HI), sexual assault, and domestic violence (DV).

If a patient presents with any psychological distress or answers yes to standard triage questions like *Do you have thoughts of harming yourself or others?* they are automatically categorized as psychiatric observation. From that moment, the protocol shifts drastically compared to the patient in the next room with abdominal pain. They're placed in a distinctive gown—at my hospital, it's green to indicate a psych admission. Other facilities use different colors: blue paper shirts and pants, purple gowns, yellow for pediatrics, you name it. The important thing is that there's always a clear distinction so staff immediately know who they're dealing with.

Once in their designated gown, psych patients are placed in a room as close to the nurses' station as possible. Why? Because this gives additional eyes, providing little room for error. I once had a patient placed in a corner room simply because we were overwhelmed and out of space. She took the hospital blanket, ripped off the threading, hid under it, and attempted to strangle herself. *Don't get too comfortable.*

They're also kept away from exit doors—another critical precaution. I've had more psych patients than I can count try to bolt from the hospital, whether to escape, smoke crack, or because they were convinced they were being chased by flying bugs. One time, a patient was placed in a bed directly across from the nurses' station—the farthest spot from the ambulance bay doors. In a split-second decision, he ripped off his EKG leads, yanked out his IV, and bolted down the long hallway toward the glowing exit sign. He punched the ambulance bay doors open and ran for it—until he tripped and landed in a bush. Never underestimate what a patient is capable of. *Never.*

The room itself also undergoes a drastic transformation. Unlike inpatient psychiatric units, EDs aren't designed with ligature-resistant settings in mind. We have machines, poles, and all sorts of equipment that get moved around without a second thought. Because of this, we have to do a little ED "feng shui" from time to time.

Every potential ligature risk or weapon must be removed. That means EKG leads, cords, blood pressure cuffs, suction tubing, thermometers, etc. are taken out. IV poles are swapped for plastic ones. Cabinets and drawers may be locked. Even food utensils are replaced with safer alternatives.

All patient clothing and personal belongings are secured in a labeled bag and stored in a designated area within the unit. Whether a patient is allowed to keep their cell phone depends on their condition and circumstances. While the general practice is to remove *all* belongings, exceptions are sometimes made based on hospital policy—always defer to your facility's guidelines. For minors, a guardian may be permitted to stay with them, but this never replaces the need for a dedicated sitter.

Now, let's talk about the sitter—because their role naturally ties into the documentation aspect of psychiatric holds. The sitter's primary responsibility is constant observation, stepping in before a patient can attempt self-harm. But as we all know, if it's not documented, it didn't happen. Sitters are tasked with Q15-minute safety checks, recording the patient's behavior (sleeping, eating, crying, etc.), and noting any restraints or restrictions. Their documentation is then scanned into the patient's chart and supported by the nurse's notes.

The nurse, of course, carries an even heavier documentation load—validating Q2H vital checks, performing Q4H mental status assessments, logging patient belongings, conducting a full head-to-toe assessment at the beginning and end of each shift (along with any additional nursing progress notes on the patient's status), administering medications as needed, and ensuring that one-to-one observation and psychiatric hold orders are renewed every twenty-four hours. I'm sure I've missed some details, but this covers the core of the workload. If the patient requires additional medical interventions, such as IV drips or restraints, the documentation responsibility increases significantly, depending on restraint type and patient age.

And that, my friends, is the full scope of psychiatric nursing care in the ED. Keep in mind that this is based on my experience and knowledge, and other hospitals may require more or different, but never less than this.

0700: Shift change.

I took over the assignment from the night nurse for an eighteen-year-old patient admitted for observation due to SI. She had voluntarily come to the emergency room the night before, reporting that she recently went through a breakup with her boyfriend of two years and was struggling academically, failing multiple classes. She expressed feelings of isolation, hopelessness, and an inability to see a future for herself. She denied any auditory or visual hallucinations, paranoia, or HI.

I glanced over at her, sitting in a green gown, looking somber. "My name is Stephanee, and I'll be your nurse today. This is Jane—she's shadowing me, so she'll be around to help with anything you need."

She was polite, looking up at us with a small smile. "Okay, sounds good."

"I know coming in here probably wasn't easy, but I want to make sure we take good care of you. Can you tell me in your own words what's been going on?" I asked, hoping to build rapport while subtly gathering the information I needed for my initial nursing note.

This wasn't just about hearing her story—I was also assessing everything beyond her words. *Was she making eye contact? Did her tone match her emotions? Did she seem withdrawn, guarded, or more open than expected?* More importantly, I was comparing what she told me to the report I had received. *Was she consistent with her story, or did she leave something out? Was she minimizing, exaggerating, or revealing more details than she had shared with the previous nurse?*

While the team already had a general idea of why she was here, my role as her nurse was to observe, document, and ensure we had the most accurate picture of her mental state. Every small detail—from her mannerisms to any discrepancies in her account—helped guide her care and the interventions we'd provide.

I listened as she recounted the same details I had already read in the chart and heard in report—her breakup, her struggles in school, the feelings of isolation and hopelessness. She spoke calmly, her tone steady, her story unchanged.

"Do you have a plan?" I asked.

Note to all nurses, regardless of your work setting or unit, the two most important behavioral health questions to ask are the following:

1. Do you have thoughts of harming yourself or others?
2. If so, do you have a plan? What is your plan?

Even if these questions have already been asked and documented by someone else, *please* ask them yourself.

She paused for a moment, then replied, "I was thinking about taking too many of my old pain pills ... Like, just enough to make everything go away."

Her answer made it clear that she remained a significant risk to herself. I nodded, keeping my voice calm. "Thank you for sharing that with me. The doctor has ordered a urine sample for you to complete in the morning. Do you need to use the bathroom now?"

She shook her head. "Not yet."

"Okay," I said, "This is Justin—he'll be your sitter today and will stay with you at all times to make sure you're safe. If you need anything, don't hesitate to let either of us know."

She nodded slightly, looking over at Justin, who gave her a kind smile.

With that, I stepped out of the room, leaving her under Justin's watch. One patient greeted, three more to go.

I made my way to my next patient—a middle-aged woman with a COPD exacerbation, her nasal cannula set at 4L, laboring slightly to breathe. She had already received steroids and a nebulizer treatment, but her O_2 sats were hovering in the low nineties. I checked her vitals, reassessed her breath sounds, and ensured her continuous pulse ox was still in place.

From there, I moved to my next room—an elderly man with altered mental status, confused and restless. His daughter sat at his bedside, anxiously wringing her hands. Labs had already been drawn, and we were awaiting results, but based on his presentation, I suspected a UTI or possibly early sepsis. I performed a quick neuro check, reoriented him as best I could, and reassured his daughter that we were closely monitoring him.

My last patient was a young man with a forehead laceration repair after a bar fight in the early hours of the morning. He was dozing off, his pain meds clearly taking effect, so I scanned through his chart, ensured his wound was still clean and dry, and left the room.

An hour had passed, and I returned to my psych patient's room to ask if she needed to use the restroom yet.

"I can get you some water," I offered.

She nodded. "Yeah, that'd be great."

As I headed to the kitchen to grab a cup of water, the morning MD pulled me aside to go over the plan of care for the laceration repair. She asked me to gather the laceration cart and all necessary supplies, then began reviewing the elderly man's urine results.

"This looks like a bad UTI," she said. "Let's make sure he has a line. I'm going to order repeat cultures and start antibiotics."

"How's the lady with COPD doing?" she asked.

"She's honestly not looking great on 4L," I admitted. "I think we should switch her to a different mask."

"Agreed," the MD said.

"I'll call RT to see if they can expedite the neb," I added.

"Sounds good. Let's also get her methylprednisolone on board."

"Already on it—I'm about to pull it now," I said.

"You're the best."

I made my way to the Pyxis, quickly navigating through the system to pull the methylprednisolone. As the machine dispensed the medication, I glanced at the clock—time was slipping away faster than I'd realized. I grabbed a flush and a syringe, then headed back toward my COPD patient's room.

As I walked down the hallway, I spotted Justin standing outside the bathroom, arms crossed, waiting patiently. His posture was relaxed. My pace slowed as I took in the scene, a small pit forming in my stomach. Something felt off.

"Everything okay?" I asked, shifting the medication into my pocket as I approached.

"Oh yeah, she's just giving the urine sample," Justin said casually.

I glanced at the door and immediately realized—it was closed.

Without hesitation, I reached for the handle and turned it.

Locked.

I noticed the change in Justin, as if he had just realized the magnitude of what this situation could mean. The panic set in for both of us, frozen in that moment, unsure of what she might be capable of behind that door. It felt as though the blood drained from our faces as reality sank in. *Oh shit. What do we do now? How do we get in?*

I knocked on the door, calling out to her, pleading for her to unlock it, but there was no answer. The key to open the door was held by security in the main lobby. Don't ask me why it was so far away for a potential emergency like this—because I'm still wondering the same thing.

Without thinking, I bolted. I sprinted down the hallway to the lobby. Thankfully, the ER isn't far from it, but even so, every second felt like an eternity. It had probably only been a minute and a half, but it felt like an hour. And in those moments, when someone is intent on hurting themselves, a minute and a half is all it takes.

There she was, standing on the toilet, trying to hang herself from the ceiling. My heart slammed against my chest as I took in the scene. It was a terrifying moment, but thankfully, there was nothing that could have allowed her to follow through.

Rule #1: Never allow a door to fully close when caring for a psychiatric patient. The line between life and death can be razor-thin, and it can be crossed in the blink of an eye. Seconds count. Always position yourself so that there is at least a foot in the doorway—yes, your foot physically wedged to prevent the door from closing completely. This gives the patient some privacy, but ensures you're still present, watching over them. Some nurses take it a step further and stand in the bathroom with the patient, never letting them out of their sight. How you manage it is up to you, but one thing is nonnegotiable: The door must never close.

Rule #2: Establish the ground rules with your sitter. Even if you've worked with someone for years, trust them, and have a great rapport, never get too comfortable. Every time, without exception, I have a conversation with my sitter about what I expect from them when it comes to patient care. I make it clear what *my* rules are for *my* patient and what my expectations are for their role. Never assume they know just because you've worked together before. Ultimately, if anything goes wrong, the responsibility falls on me. I'm the nurse. I'm responsible for the care of my patient, and the sitter is working under my direction. And don't forget—this conversation needs to be charted too. If it isn't documented, it didn't happen. Always remember: The buck stops with you. So take the time to dot your i's and cross your t's.

Rule #3: Learn to balance trust and caution. As nurses, especially when working with psychiatric patients, we walk this delicate balance every day. There's a fine line between trusting a patient's words and being cautious about their actions. For example, when a patient answers questions like *Do you feel safe at home?* or *Do you have thoughts of hurting yourself or others?* we *have* to trust their answers. Shit, I met you five minutes ago, and I have no reason not to take your word! But there are times when we must trust their words but not their actions. It's like saying, *I believe what you're telling me, but I can't trust what you might do.*

And it's not out of malice; it's rooted in compassion and responsibility. The reality is that nurses are responsible for your well-being. Psychiatric illness can distort a patient's perception of reality, and we can't ignore that.

I want to keep my patients safe and see them overcome these challenges. And sometimes, that means doing things they won't like. It means invading their space, taking their belongings, questioning their every move—not because I want to, but because I care. The weight of their safety is on me. And that responsibility will never be ignored for as long as you're a competent nurse.

So lead with compassion, validate their feelings, be their anchor when their world feels chaotic. But never lose sight of the fact that your first priority is their safety not their comfort.

Code Gold ...?

Do you ever have those moments at work where you just look around and think, *No way is this real life?* Or you find yourself laughing because you're half convinced someone's playing a prank on you, like you're on an episode of *Punk'd?* Like the time a grown man came in with a living hamster lodged up his ass. Or the inmate who "couldn't pee," only to discover he had a rubber band wrapped around his penis to hide weapons in jail but instead was cutting off his circulation. And let's not forget the time the hospital was being hacked for weeks, and we had to switch to paper charting—imagine an emergency department using paper charting during a code. You glance around at your coworkers, their expressions worthy of an episode of *The Office*. Because honestly, some of these situations are straight out of a sitcom.

There I was, huddled in the med room with my fellow nurses, frantically googling *What is a Code Gold?*

But let's back up a bit. EDs vary in size, but they typically have multiple nurse "pods" scattered throughout the unit. If you're assigned to beds near the ambulance bay, you'll likely spend most of your time at the nearest nurse pod. The same goes for the middle and back sections of the ER. Physicians follow a similar pattern—while they have a designated physician's room, usually near the trauma bay, they tend to spread out across the department, working from computers in different pods. Occasionally, they'll retreat to their room for discussions or a quick break when things slow down.

This collaborative environment is one of the things I love most about the ER. We work side by side—literally—at the pods, fostering a sense of unity and mutual respect despite the hierarchy. Physicians hear our chatter, witness our patient interactions firsthand, and genuinely value our input. It's this dynamic that makes the ER feel less like a workplace and more like a well-oiled, chaotic yet deeply connected family.

Another day, another wave of patients crammed into every possible space—doubled up in rooms, lining the hallways, and spilling into chairs. Just when I thought I'd seen the ER at its most chaotic, the universe said, *Hold my beer.*

That day, I was assigned to the beds in the "back" of the unit. Being farther from the ambulance bay, this area is typically designated for lower-acuity patients—but don't let that fool you. We're still managing diabetic ketoacidosis (DKA) insulin drips, conscious sedations, sepsis, and more. The only difference? This isn't where you'll find the trauma cases— no gunshot wounds, massive car accidents, Code Blues, or hemorrhages.

Naturally, I gravitated toward the back nurse pod, where seven computers sat—six occupied by nurses, and one forever reserved for the physician covering that section.

In the hall, diagonally across from the nurses' station, sat an intoxicated man sobering up. He was visibly agitated but kept to himself. Since the start of my shift, he hadn't caused any trouble—and since he wasn't my patient, I focused on my own assignments, tending to my own patients.

I walked back to the nurses' station, hoping to catch up on my charting. The morning had been nonstop, and I was scrambling to get up to speed with nearly every one of my patients. I settled into the computer next to the physician's usual spot, which was empty since he was in a nearby room with a patient. I could hear his voice but couldn't make out the conversation.

A few moments later, I caught his figure in my peripheral vision. I looked up, and he met my gaze. In a firm but controlled voice, careful not to draw attention, he said, "Call a Code Gold."

It took me a moment to process what he was asking. Not because I didn't understand or was incapable of doing so, but because I had a genuine thought: *What the fuck is a Code Gold?*

In all my years of nursing—across multiple hospitals, job positions, and enough shifts to rewire my brain chemistry—I had never heard of this particular color-coded emergency. And listen, hospitals love their codes. There's a whole damn rainbow of them. Code Blue? Arrest. Code Red? Fire. Code Silver? Active shooter. But Code Gold? That was new.

The doctor stared at me, waiting. His face was serious, firm, as if I should know exactly what to do. Oh God. Am I supposed to know what this is? Should I know what to do? I've been doing this long enough … How do I not know what this is? My brain was running through every possible scenario. Meanwhile, my actual body was sitting completely frozen in my chair, blinking at him with the mental response time of a sedated patient on Versed.

Not wanting to look like a complete idiot, I turned—very subtly, so as not to alert him—to the nurses at the station.

"The doctor wants to call a Code Gold."

Silence.

Then the slow realization that I was not the only one confused.

I glanced at one nurse. *What the fuck?* was written all over her face.

Another nurse, completely unbothered, continued charting like nothing happened.

Another let out a deep, exhausted sigh, as if this were the final straw in a very long day of nonsense.

And then, in perfect harmony, they all said: "What's a Code Gold?"

Oh, thank God. It wasn't just me.

Now, normally when we call a code, we just dial the operator and say, "Call Code [Insert Known Code Here]," and they handle the rest. Simple. Efficient.

The confusion spread quickly. Nurses started whispering to each other.

"Do you know what a Code Gold is?"

"Never heard of it."

"Did we just make this up?"

"Are we about to summon something?"

I gravitated toward a few coworkers, and without a word, we all silently shuffled into the med room, like a group of high schoolers with their besties when drama was unfolding. Phones were out in seconds, each of us frantically googling hospital code colors like our careers depended on it.

Nothing.

The longer we stalled, the worse it looked. We needed to act before the doctor realized we were collectively too scared to ask. So in a moment of quiet resignation, we caved and called the operator.

"Code Gold?" the operator repeated, audibly confused.

Trust me, girl, we are just as confused as you are, but just go with it, okay?

And then, over the loudspeaker:

"Code Gold, ER. Code Gold, ER."

The moment it echoed through the hospital, you could *see* the confusion ripple outward.

Security guards, mid-step, suddenly slowed down, looking up as if the answer might be written in the ceiling tiles. Nurses paused in their tasks, their faces scrunched in uncertainty. Even a passing Environmental Services (EVS) worker stopped pushing his mop, eyes narrowing slightly as if to say, *Now what in the hell is that?*

I peered out of the med room, trying to assess the damage. The charge nurse stood at the station, head tilted upward, eyes scanning the room like she was waiting for divine intervention to explain what had just been summoned.

We had officially called a Code Gold.

Now ... someone just needed to tell us what it meant.

Nobody said anything after that. We silently carried on with our nursing duties, pretending that we weren't the ones who had called the strange code overhead. A few moments of awkward silence passed, and then it was back to the chaos of the ER.

Until about fifteen minutes later, the doctor strolled up to me, looking embarrassed. He cleared his throat. "I am so sorry. I didn't mean to call it a Code Gold," he said, his voice low and apologetic. "I meant a Code Gray for the patient in the hall. He was being really mouthy and kept trying to take pictures of me, so I wanted security to come over. So sorry, that's what we call it at my other hospital!"

And just like that, the confusion lifted. We had all spent the last fifteen minutes in a state of complete panic over nothing—well, not nothing, but definitely not a "Code Gold." In hindsight, it was hilarious. I couldn't stop laughing for the next few hours, and neither could the rest of the team. We were all so lost, but somehow, we'd just run with it, riding that wave of chaos like we were born for it. I mean ... fake it till you make it, right?

The ER can be a tough, high-pressure environment, but it's those little inside jokes and moments of genuine camaraderie that make it all worthwhile. You have to lean into the teamwork, or the job can wear you down. And when you can collaborate, laugh, and enjoy each other's company? That's when you know you've hit the jackpot of a team.

From that point on, every time I worked with that doctor, we'd joke to each other, "Call Code Gold." Because those moments of shared absurdity? They're worth more than gold.

A Cinderella Story

A thirty-five-year-old male presented to the ER with an episode of syncope at work. No warning, no witnesses. He said it "happened out of nowhere."

"This ever happen before?" the physician asked.

"No."

"Any chest pain or pressure?"

"No."

"Shortness of breath?"

"No."

"Did you hit your head?"

"I don't think so."

"Allergies?"

"No."

"Recreational drugs?"

"No."

"Do you smoke?"

"Yes."

The physician pulled the stethoscope from one ear. "You're young. Stop now."

His EKG showed a cardiac arrhythmia—nothing immediately life-threatening but enough to warrant further workup.

A nine-year-old girl arrived with her mother and father. The mother was frantic, her panic filling the room before the words even left her mouth. The child had been leaning on her bedroom windowsill when the window screen suddenly gave way, sending her tumbling two stories onto the lawn.

By some miracle, she had landed on grass. No obvious deformities, no loss of consciousness—but a fall like that wasn't something to brush off. A full neurologic exam, scans, and a pediatric trauma consult were already in motion.

The shift pressed on in a blur—minor traumas, cardioversions, EtOH (drunk patients). The usual.

Until the dispatch phone rang.

Some hospitals call it dispatch, the red phone, the red line, encodes, doc-in-a-box, radio report— you name it. It sits far from the standard hospital phones and never fails to scare the shit out of me with the loudest sound known to humankind. Essentially, it's a phone dedicated solely to EMS runs en route to the hospital. The ambulance crew calls in, gives a short and quick background on the patient, explains what's been done, provides an ETA, and relays any other pertinent information.

The call lasts no more than a minute or two, but in that time, whoever answers must relay the information to the right people: the physician, charge nurse, operator to call a code overhead, respiratory to prepare for an incoming arrest or distress, and so on. Depending on the hospital's setup, the call might come directly from EMS or through a dispatch center acting as the middleman. Either way, the information is live, and immediate preparation is required.

"Level 1 trauma, ETA three minutes. Thirty-two-year-old male. Motorcycle versus semi. CPR in progress."

Three minutes to prepare.

And to be honest, three minutes is a long time—an eternity, even.

It's hard to explain the feeling of unpredictability in the ER, what goes on in your head as those three minutes tick by. The racing thoughts of what you might see, how right or wrong you are in your guesses, the mental run-through of random protocols just to calm your mind and reassure yourself that you know what you're doing. That feeling becomes a constant in a nurse's life—though it's not the kind of constant you particularly ask for. It just comes with the job, and you learn to rewire your brain to embrace it.

Because at 1100, you could be peacefully putting fresh sheets on a discharged patient's gurney. And at 1101, you hear the blood-curdling screams of a mother running through the doors, clutching her two-year-old daughter—her face torn apart by a dog attack.

There is nothing—nothing outside those hospital walls—that compares.

The team fell into position, like a well-oiled machine. I, the primary nurse, stood at the computer, waiting for the full breakdown from EMS, with the physician nearby, hands on hips, mentally running through every possible scenario. The scribe grabbed the nearest piece of paper—wrinkled, stained, it didn't matter—and prepared to jot down everything: code times, meds given, CPR cycles, shocks, IVs.

The IV starters were already assembling their supplies, hands steady with the anticipation of what's to come. The med pushers hovered near the crash cart, prepped with epi, bicarb, and whatever else we might need. The CPR duo stretched their arms, mentally preparing to rotate in. The supply grabbers, the AED monitors—every single person in that room had a job, and every job mattered.

Gowns on. Gloves tight.

The room was charged with a controlled urgency.

And now, here we were, nearing the end of our three minutes when lights and sirens pulled up, doors swinging open. *1311.* The stretcher rolled in, the EMS team just behind it.

"Thirty-two-year-old male," the EMS crew called out, wheeling the patient to the bedside. "Collided with a semi-truck. Motorcycle tire lodged in the truck bed, sent him flying through traffic. GCS four, unconscious, possible head trauma. He's been down for a while—PEA on scene, ROSC after one round of epi in the field, coded again en route, two more rounds of epi. Still bagging. No response to noxious stimuli. Positive Grey Turner's sign. Severe deformities and abrasions noted along the left arm and leg. IV access—18G in the right forearm, IO in the right tibia with blood return."

The team didn't need to be told twice. A nurse was already cutting away the patient's clothes, exposing the mangled body underneath. Each movement was deliberate, swift—the clock ticking louder with every second that passed. The AED pads were placed on the chest, and the monitor beeped loudly, showing a flatline—asystole. The physician looked over, assessing the situation, already calculating the next steps.

"Let's get our leads on him, run a BP. I want to see this on the monitor. Resume chest compressions. Let's see how he responds to another one of epi," the physician ordered, his voice low but firm, never faltering.

Another nurse grabbed the vial, pushed the dose, and simultaneously called out, "One milligram epi given!"

1mg epi @ 1314, the scribe wrote down.

As the team moved with a synchrony honed by countless hours of practice, the scribe frantically documented everything heard, seen, and done. Her notes acted as a second witness to my real-time charting, and once the scene settled, I would rely on her scribbles to fill in the gaps of what I might have missed.

Amid the movement, RT took over at the head of the bed, smoothly placing the endotracheal tube (ET) to secure the airway.

"7.5 ET, 27 at the lip."

7.5 ET, 27 @ left side lip @ 1315, the scribe wrote down.

The patient's chest heaved under the pressure of CPR, the compressions deep and steady; a third nurse simultaneously prepped another IV line.

"Sixteen right AC, going for blood draw."

A fourth nurse called out, "Blood gases drawn."

16G R AC; labs & ABGs drawn @ 1315, the scribe noted.

A fifth nurse wheeled the rapid infuser closer—prepped with fluids and blood bags. His life was slipping away, unmistakably, but we kept working.

The extended focus assessment with sonography in trauma (E-FAST) machine was brought to the bedside. An attending took a breath and slid the ultrasound probe over the patient's abdomen. The image flickered on the screen. Free fluid—hemoperitoneum. He didn't need to say it out loud; his face said it all.

"Trauma surgery is on the way. We need to stabilize him for transfer," he said, his eyes still on the screen. "He's bleeding, but we can work with this. Let's start MTP."

The blood products began to flow into the patient's veins—eight units packed red blood cells (PRBC) and four fresh frozen plasma (FFP), to be exact. The scribe noted all units and times administered.

"Two-minute pulse check!" the scribe shouted, allowing a moment for the staff to rotate on CPR and check a rhythm. We held our breath—silence so loud.

No pulse. Asystole.

1316 pulse check; absent. Rhythm: asystole, the scribe scribbled.

"Push one more epi," the physician said, turning to the team. "We're going to need more volume. Get that pressure up, keep the compressions going."

"Got it," I replied, checking the monitor once more. "Fluids and blood are moving in."

"One milligram epi given!" the nurse shouted.

1mg epi @ 1317. The scribe's pen scratched across the paper, documenting each action, each medication given.

"Two-minute pulse check!" the scribe shouted again.

Hands came off the chest. Silence. Eyes staring into space as the mind raced. Fingers pressed against various pulse points, desperately searching for even the faintest beat.

No pulse. Asystole.

1318 pulse check; absent. Rhythm: asystole.

The cycle repeated. And repeated. And repeated. For twelve more minutes. Each minute that passed pulled him farther from life as we desperately tried to reel him back in. Another minute we prayed he wouldn't bleed out completely. Another minute of last-ditch efforts.

As a health care professional, the decision to stop is never taken lightly—because deep down, it can feel like a surrender, and that's something painfully hard to accept. But nestled within the thought of surrender is a flicker of hope, a thin thread of possibility urging you to keep going. Maybe, in the next ten seconds, we'll feel a pulse. Maybe, in the next moment, a miracle will unfold before us. The *what-if* gnaws at you. *What if* we pushed just one more epi? *What if* we kept the compressions going a little longer? We've seen it work before, and while it doesn't always go our way, that one time is enough to make us believe it could happen again.

Another two minutes passed. The scribe called it again. "Pulse check!"

"I think I have one."

A split second of hesitation. Then—"Confirm it."

Another set of hands joined, pressing firmly against cooling skin. A hush fell over the room, the only sound the mechanical whir of the ventilator cycling air into his lungs.

A single, sluggish thump beneath fingertips.

"Yup, I feel it. It's faint, but I feel it."

The energy in the room shifted, subtle but undeniable. The physician leaned forward, his gaze flicking between the monitor and the body on the table. "We're not out of the woods yet, but we're not giving up."

The momentum picked up again, but this time, it carried something else with it—the flicker of hope.

I watched as the physician walked past, his voice barely above a whisper. "Cinderella."

Against all odds, we achieved return of spontaneous circulation (ROSC)—and it stayed that way. The patient was rushed to emergency surgery to address a grade III liver laceration and grade IV kidney laceration, which had caused internal bleeding that dumped half of his blood supply into the abdominal cavity and out his Foley catheter. He received over fifty units of blood and FFP during his stay, carefully titrated on epinephrine, ketamine, Neo-Synephrine, and vasopressin in the ICU. Diagnostics revealed a hemopneumothorax, right parietal intracranial bleed, and T1–T3 spinal fractures, along with numerous other broken bones. Subsequent surgeries reconstructed his shattered right arm and leg, and his recovery would be long and grueling. But yes, he did recover—physically and neurologically. With months of PT/OT, he reintegrated back into life, piece by piece.

Some would call it a Cinderella story—the same words the physician mumbled under his breath as we achieved ROSC.

And you're probably wondering, *What the fuck does that mean? Who's Cinderella?*

In medicine, a Cinderella story refers to an outcome that defies all odds. It's that rare moment when a patient, against every probability, survives or makes an incredible recovery from a situation deemed deadly—when you stand there thinking, *There's no feasible way this patient will recover in a meaningful way.* Like Cinderella, who rose from the lowest of lows to a fairy-tale ending, these patients start in devastation, facing countless disadvantages, yet somehow, through the relentless efforts of the medical team, they pull through. It's the kind of miracle that doesn't happen every day, but when it does, you know you've witnessed something extraordinary.

This patient—a true Cinderella story. And for all the patients who come in with the most tragic cases, knocking on death's door, we hope they'll have a Cinderella story of their own.

I've only heard this saying twice in my career. *Twice.* A testament to its rarity.

The first time I encountered it was when a woman walked into the ER, presenting a set of symptoms that immediately raised red flags. She was in her mid-forties and reported chest pain radiating down her left arm, accompanied by nausea and lightheadedness. These symptoms had been ongoing for the past week, but when I asked about them, she explained that she had written it off as indigestion from the greasy hamburger she'd eaten the night before.

She had hoped the discomfort would pass, but as the days went by, the symptoms only grew more persistent. It wasn't until the nausea became unbearable, and the dizziness and weakness left her struggling to get out of bed, that she realized she could no longer ignore it. Reluctantly, she called her husband to take her to the ER.

Heart attack, as you might've guessed.

The team rushed in, activating the Code STEMI protocol, and she was whisked away to the Cath lab. She survived the unsurvivable—a 100 percent occlusion of the left anterior descending artery known as the *widowmaker*. Named for its high fatality rate and the spouses it so often leaves behind.

Cinderella story.

A week later, she returned with chest pressure—as a precaution. She was okay, though understandably shaken after surviving a widowmaker days earlier.

"I counted nine people in my room last time," she told me, "but for some reason, I only remember you. Thank you for saving my life."

Some stories linger long after the shift ends—not because they were expected, but because they weren't. They catch us off guard, redefine what we thought we knew, and leave us reflecting on the delicate balance between medicine and mystery.

They can stir something deep in us: hope, faith, awe. They remind us why we do what we do—why we fight for each patient, why we double-check labs at 3 a.m., why we push for that extra test when something "doesn't quite add up." They are the exceptions that reaffirm the value of vigilance and the power of timing, teamwork, and perseverance.

Yet they also carry a quiet burden.

Cinderella stories are, by definition, rare. And when they happen, they can set unrealistic expectations for future outcomes. Families may hold tightly to the belief that their loved one will be the exception too. Providers may feel pressure to recreate the impossible. And sometimes, when the outcome isn't miraculous, it can feel like a failure—even when everything was done right.

In my own practice, I've learned to hold space for both: the reality of evidence-based medicine and the rare, remarkable story that defies it. Cinderella stories should not drive our protocols, but they do shape our humanity. They ask us to remain open to possibility without becoming blinded by it. They remind us that while science is our guide, compassion is our constant—and that our purpose is not to chase miracles but to practice in a way that honors the possibility of one.

The Lesson Isn't
in the Outcome

It was a Sunday afternoon when a patient walked into the ER with a chief complaint of generalized weakness and poor appetite, symptoms he'd been experiencing for several days. He was visiting a close friend from out of state and mentioned that he "just hadn't been feeling well since arriving." To give you some context, he was in his mid-thirties, denied any comorbidities, and otherwise appeared well. Strangely, he had chosen to come to the ER rather than urgent care.

Upon initial examination, I found him to be tachypneic—his breathing was rapid and shallow. His skin felt cold to the touch, to the point that I had trouble obtaining an oxygen saturation reading on his finger. He mentioned feeling dehydrated due to his poor appetite and lack of adequate fluid intake. My critical thinking kicked in: *Could dehydration be the reason he felt so cold?* The triage nurse placed him in my bed, and I immediately hooked him up to the monitor and drew labs.

Remember: *line, labs, EKG*—the classic ER intervention trio that should *always* be your starting point.

While waiting for his lab results, I decided to start with the basics. Since he complained of dehydration, I hung a liter of fluids, hoping it would help him feel a little better.

As I worked, he chatted about his trip. He was from Michigan and spoke warmly of his wife, whom he described as lovely. He shared that he was in California for his best friend's bachelor party—a close friendship spanning nearly a decade. Rather than a wild night out, they had opted for a relaxed coastal trip.

As he spoke, I monitored his vitals. His blood pressure was slightly low, his heart rate slightly high—but nothing alarming. We had no baseline to compare it to, so I made a mental note to keep an eye on them.

Still, he was alert and oriented, speaking in full, clear sentences. He wasn't in any visible distress—just kept repeating that he felt *off* this weekend. Nothing about him screamed critical. I assumed we'd get his labs back, give him some fluids, and figure out what was going on.

I sat down at the nurses' station to catch up on charting, the steady hum of the ER around me: monitors beeping, a few coworkers laughing at a YouTube video, the secretary juggling phone calls. In the background, I could hear the physicians talking among themselves.

"This guy shouldn't be alive right now."

My eyes flicked up from my screen. My brain started ticking through the list of patients in the ER, trying to place who they were talking about. (One thing about ER nurses: We're nosy by nature. It's just part of who we are. Even when I'm off the clock, minding my own business at the grocery store, I find myself sneaking peeks at the active ambulance, curious about what's happening inside.)

Not my patient. Couldn't be.

I went back to my work, flipping through unmarked tasks, checking the waiting room queue.

Then my work phone buzzed.

MD: This guy is really sick. We need to admit him ASAP.

I blinked, my mind racing. *What?*

Then … the new results icon popped up on his chart.

I clicked.

White blood cells: **32,000/mm³**

Lactate: **13.9 mmol/L**

pH: **7.12**

Bicarbonate (HCO_3^-): **12 mEq/L**

Creatinine: **4.6 mg/dL**

BUN: **58 mg/dL**

At the root of it all? Cholecystitis—an inflamed gallbladder. But this wasn't just any routine case. It had likely gone untreated for too long, and by the time he arrived in the ER, it had spiraled into severe sepsis, metabolic acidosis, and acute renal failure. In other words, his inflamed gallbladder had set off a chain reaction, slowly shutting down his organs one by one.

The MD came up behind me, and we exchanged a look as if we both just knew. He leaned in and said, "This guy should not be alive right now. Your job is to keep him alive for the next ten hours. And I'll be very impressed if he makes it."

I felt an instant wave of pressure settle on my chest. Usually, doctors maintain a certain level of calm in situations like this. Even in critical cases, they give off a still confidence that we, as nurses, can tap into. But not this time.

This time, the doctor looked worried.

And when a physician starts to freak out, I start to freak out—because in this hierarchy, they're the ones we look to for reassurance.

For the next ten hours, I never left that room. I watched him like a hawk, learning new nursing skills along the way. I assisted with placing a temporary dialysis port at the bedside for emergent dialysis and managed an extensive sepsis protocol. I titrated his drips and learned how to communicate life-threatening news to a patient who thought he was going to return to his friend's bachelor party in a few hours.

Luckily, he made it through those ten hours—and days later, walked out of the ICU a healthy man, able to return home to his wife in Michigan.

The following day, yet again, another man in his mid-thirties walked into the ER, complaining of feeling "under the weather." He attributed it mostly to a cold, mentioning a productive cough that had been lingering for a few days along with general malaise. His skin appeared slightly pale, and his overall demeanor exuded exhaustion as I assessed him. "Of all the days you've been sick, what made you come in *today*?" I asked.

A helpful tip: When patients present to the ER with long-standing complaints—especially those that have lasted for weeks and it's unclear why they didn't seek care sooner—ask, "What made you come in *today*, of all days?" This question often uncovers the true chief complaint—the factor that prompted them to seek help *at that specific moment.* This principle also applies when a patient lists a multitude of complaints. If they mention several concerns, I'll ask, "Out of everything that's bothering you, what is the main issue that led you to come in *today*?" Essentially, it helps organize their complaints by priority, pinpointing what is bothering them the *most* that drove them to seek care *now.*

In this case, he said his shortness of breath wouldn't resolve—it was "annoying" and made it difficult to perform his normal daily tasks. During triage, his vital signs were mostly within normal limits, aside from a slightly elevated heart rate.

Behind the scenes, my mind was already running through a mental checklist. Based on his symptoms and the fact that it was flu season, I initially suspected a viral infection—something like the flu or a common cold. Nine times out of ten, patients with similar complaints would test positive for influenza.

But like I always say, we build mental file cabinets over time—structured ways of thinking, boxes to check, possible scenarios to consider, and body systems that may be involved. You develop a spectrum of best-case and worst-case scenarios because (1) anticipating the worst is what saves lives, and (2) the "worst" does not discriminate.

In a worst-case scenario, my mind went to a potential pulmonary embolism—a blood clot that had traveled to his lungs, causing his shortness of breath. Is this dramatic? Well, yes. But a possibility? Absolutely. Our job was to systematically rule possibilities in or out through lab work, flu swabs, and other diagnostics.

As he was being wheeled back to one of my beds, he suddenly began to vomit profusely. My coworker and I quickly placed him on the monitor, and shortly after, he had a syncopal episode. Minutes later, as if in a rapid cascade of events, he went into cardiac arrest.

Much like the day prior, I never left that room. We spent six long hours doing everything in our power to keep this patient alive. He was a husband, a father, and a kind soul who didn't deserve the hand he had been dealt. I monitored every one of his vitals, carefully titrating all of his drips. I held his hand and spoke to his wife, sharing what a great man he was.

It was traumatic, sudden—and despite all our efforts, he passed away a few hours later. We couldn't pinpoint the exact cause of his sudden cardiac arrest. The doctor on shift that day speculated he may have suffered from viral cardiomyopathy, which led to myocarditis—an inflammation of the heart. This condition weakens the heart's ability to pump blood effectively, ultimately leading to heart failure.

That's the theory, though we couldn't confirm it for certain.

There's no blatant medical lesson to be learned from these two outcomes, no point in the story where I can say, *Always remember these symptoms for xyz*, or tell you to know your lab value ranges. Because the lesson isn't in the outcome—it's in the act of showing up, giving your best, and understanding that some things are simply beyond your control.

Sometimes, you get to be part of a miracle. Other times, no matter how well you do your job, it just doesn't work out that way. Some people will live, and some won't. You have no control over that. All you can do is show up, do your job, and keep going.

We do our best to find answers, but medicine isn't always black and white. Illness and death don't follow rules, nor do they owe us explanations. The contrast between these two patients—same age, similar complaints, yet vastly different outcomes—serves as a sobering reminder that life is fragile, unpredictable, and often unfair. As nurses, we are not in the business of guaranteeing survival; we are in the business of giving people their best possible chance at survival. And sometimes, the most meaningful thing we can do is simply bear witness—to fight for them, to stand by them, and to make sure they are seen, no matter the outcome. *That* is the lesson.

The Trust We Earn

Your nurse is skillfully trained to recognize even the most subtle changes in your baseline—details that could mean the difference between life and death, in the bluntest terms. Trust their expertise, listen to their guidance, and know that their priority is your well-being.

Let me tell you a story. A young man—if I remember correctly, in his late twenties—was wheeled into the ER by a friend. He was AOx4 but covered in blood, with multiple lacerations on his forehead, nose, and hands. He stated that he had fallen while leaving the airport, hit his head, but denied losing consciousness. We transferred him onto a gurney, and I began a series of assessment questions.

"Can you tell me what happened in your own words?"

"I was running to catch my ride after my flight, tripped over the curb, and face-planted—just went straight down."

"And just to confirm, you don't remember losing consciousness?"

"No, I know for sure I didn't."

"What happened right after the fall?"

Asking about the moments before and after the fall helps further confirm that he didn't experience syncope. Sometimes, patients will answer no to one question but yes to the same question when phrased differently. This is our way of ensuring we gather the most accurate details about our biggest concerns.

"I remember thinking, *Damn, that was a hard fall,* but I just turned over and laid there for a second. Someone came up and asked if I needed help getting up."

"Do you have any blurry vision?"

"Slightly."

"Double vision?"

"No."

"Numbness or tingling anywhere?"

"No."

"Nausea or dizziness?"

"No, not really."

"Any vomiting on the way here?"

"No."

"Any sensitivity to the light in this room?"

"No, I'm good."

"Can you tell me where your pain is?"

"My head hurts near all the cuts—my nose too, obviously. My arms kind of hurt from bracing the fall, and that's about it."

"How would you describe the pain?"

"Just a throbbing pain. Not sharp, more deep and dull. Probably like a five out of ten."

As he answered, I continued my assessment, listening to his words while simultaneously evaluating him objectively. With experience, these two assessments become second nature, happening simultaneously and with increasing speed over time. *Does he seem dazed or confused? Can he follow simple instructions and answer my questions appropriately? How is his range of motion? Is his speech clear and coherent? Are his pupils equal in size and reactive to light?* All of these assessments were stored away in my mental "head injury/fall" file cabinet.

As I finished the assessment with the standard screening questions, I glanced toward the door and made eye contact with an EMT.

"Could you grab me a C-collar?" I asked.

With any head injury or fall, the standard of care is to apply a C-collar until imaging can rule out potential neck or spine injuries. While the patient hadn't complained of neck or back pain, and his fall had been from ground level without any loss of consciousness, he was no different in my eyes and still required a C-collar. It reminded me of the patient with the late-onset allergic reaction. You remember her, right? The one with the love note from the doctor—ew, all right, moving on. Despite her complaints seeming minimal and her repeatedly dismissing her shortness of breath, we made the decision to keep her overnight as a precaution. In the end, that cautious decision ended up saving her life.

While these "overly cautious protocols" may sometimes seem inconvenient or unnecessary, they are grounded in our experience—experience you may not yet have or may never encounter in your lifetime. Yes, that's a blessing in disguise for the general public, who don't have to live with the constant *what-ifs* that we face. But we've seen things that highlight the importance of not overlooking even the smallest details. And just like that, one C-collar coming up!

"Wait, hold on," he said, his brow furrowing. "Why do I need a C-collar? I don't have any neck pain."

I paused and looked his way, already knowing where this was headed. The tone in his voice told me he was about to complain about wearing the C-collar. I could already predict the conversation and prepared myself to explain it multiple times.

"It's standard practice," I said, maintaining a calm tone. "We need to stabilize your neck and spine until we can rule out any injuries. Even if you're not feeling pain there, we still have to take precautions."

The EMT returned with the C-collar, placing it gently around the patient's neck and lowering the bed to adhere to protocol. The patient shifted, clearly uncomfortable. "This is ridiculous," he muttered.

"I know it's not fun, but once we get the scans and results, we can take this off. I won't leave it on for any longer than necessary."

"It's not even necessary *now*," he said, rolling his eyes and glancing at his friend, who was chuckling in the corner at how silly he looked with the C-collar on.

For two hours, he complained—rightfully so, in a way. Those things are incredibly uncomfortable. But in another way, he was rather disrespectful, making rude remarks, questioning my care, and mumbling under his breath. And I can say that without any remorse now because he can thank his lucky stars that we pushed for his safety. C4 neck fracture. Yup, you heard that right.

It happens all the time. If you're a nurse, you've heard it. The comments, the questioning, the unsolicited suggestions about how to do our jobs. Patients—sometimes out of fear, sometimes out of skepticism, and sometimes just out of habit—question our expertise more than they accept it.

We don't need a thank you. We don't expect it. Most of the time, we're just another face in a long blurry hospital stay. But what we do expect—what we should expect—is respect.

Respect for the years of education, the clinical training, and the thousands of hours spent at the bedside that allows us to make critical decisions. Respect for the fact that when we say you need that C-collar, it's not just a suggestion—it's the result of training, experience, and a deep-rooted understanding of what can go wrong. Respect for the fact that when we place that IV, it's not luck—it's skill. And respect for the fact that when we explain your condition, your treatment, or your next steps, we carry the knowledge to do so.

More often than not, though, what we get instead are the jabs—the subtle (and not-so-subtle) digs at our competence. The patient who scoffs at our lengthy assessment. The one who rolls their eyes at our precautions. The backhanded compliment: *Wow, I'm surprised you got that IV on the first try,* as if we don't place dozens of them a day. The *Have you ever done this before?* or *Do you know what you're doing?* as if our ability is up for debate. The *Do you really need to take that much blood?* or worse, *Didn't you go to nursing school?*—as if my education needs to be validated before I can care for you. The *I don't need that,* or *Well, last time they did it this way,* because somehow, their last hospital visit holds more weight than our current clinical judgment.

And yet when I say, *You need that C-collar*, I mean it. Not because I want to inconvenience you, not because it's protocol for protocol's sake, but because I've seen what happens when we don't. In the end, those little moments of doubt don't shake our confidence. We know why we're here. We know what we're doing. And when our gut says, *This isn't just a simple fall*, we listen.

Even if you don't.

It's like a sixth sense—developed over years of experience and sharpened by countless moments of paying attention to the smallest details. One of the most valuable skills a nurse can develop is intuition. Think of the nurse who parks the crash cart outside a patient's room because they *just have a gut feeling.*

I remember a case involving a thirteen-month-old infant brought in by their parents for vomiting and fever that began one day ago. During my initial assessment, I noticed a faint-yellow hue to the baby's skin—so subtle that anyone else might have questioned my judgment. And they did. "I don't see that at all, that's crazy." "Can you focus on the actual issue here?" The parents were more concerned about the vomiting and fever, but my intuition told me something else was at play. I couldn't shake the feeling, so I pushed for additional lab work. The parents were understandably hesitant, skeptical about any procedure that might seem unnecessary. As a rule, we always strive to be as noninvasive as possible, especially with pediatric patients who don't fully understand the purpose behind the discomfort.

The lab results came back with an alarmingly high alanine aminotransferase (ALT) level of 3,168 U/L. For context, the normal range for ALT in pediatric patients is typically between 7–55 U/L for males and 7–45 U/L for females. Such an elevated value could indicate serious conditions, including bone cancer, cholecystitis (gallbladder inflammation), cirrhosis (liver inflammation), or hepatocarcinoma (the aggressive cancer my mother had)—conditions that are exceptionally rare in a thirteen-month-old child, but this discovery ultimately altered the trajectory of her life.

All of this to say, trust in the years we've dedicated to being at your bedside, in the education that brought us here, and in the experience that enables us to make critical decisions.

And to the patients, families, and loved ones reading this, this part is for you: I understand that trust is earned, and I know it comes with stipulations—because sometimes, we are wrong. Sometimes the health care system fails you.

My own mother was failed by this system—and I grew up watching it happen. For nearly a decade, she sought answers—earnestly, patiently—in a system that continuously dismissed her concerns. Each time she spoke up, she was met with oversimplified explanations: a gluten intolerance, a new workout regimen, stress. When her symptoms persisted and her intuition told her something wasn't right, she was told she was overthinking it.

"I'd like to refer you to a psychiatrist," one physician told her. "Because there's nothing physically wrong with you."

But there was.

She was right all along. By the time a tumor the size of a golf ball was discovered on her ovary, it was too late. Years had passed without a diagnosis—years in which someone could have caught it, should have listened. But no one did.

For a long time, I carried a deep, searing anger. I resented the health care professionals who had failed her—the ones who were supposed to advocate, to protect, to care. I despised the system for what it took from her. From me.

Until I became part of it.

And stepping into that world didn't erase my grief or dull my rage, but it gave me clarity.

It revealed just how broken the system truly is—but also how much potential it still holds. I saw the burnout that quietly chips away at empathy, the policies that prioritize numbers over nuance, and the well-meaning professionals who are just trying to keep their heads above water.

I came to realize that it isn't always cruelty or carelessness that leads to failure.

Sometimes, it's fatigue.

Sometimes, it's tunnel vision.

Sometimes, it's a system that forces providers to choose between thoroughness and survival.

That doesn't excuse it.

It doesn't make it right.

But it gave me insight.

It helped me understand that, while the system failed my mom, many of the people within it never wanted that outcome. And because of what I lived through, I can understand where your skepticism in our decisions and care stems from.

Still, we're human too. And while we strive for excellence, we don't always get it right.

But most of us? We care deeply about what we do. We love our work, even when it's tough, and we don't take your trust for granted. Yes, occasionally, you may encounter a nurse or physician who is far past their prime, burned out, or just not where they should be in their career. Unfortunately, those individuals give the entire system a bad name. But that's not reflective of the profession as a whole. We do our best to serve you well.

So while we're not perfect, we show up every day trying to do better. And we hope you can find it in you to trust the years of training, experience, and heart we put into our work—because it's our *privilege* to care for you.

The Paradox

Nursing is a profession of paradoxes. In one breath, you can feel completely emptied—your body aching, your mind overloaded, your heart numb from witnessing too much. And in the next, you're laughing with a patient, celebrating a small win, or sharing a quiet moment of connection that reminds you why you started this in the first place. The truth is, burnout and joy don't exist at opposite ends of a spectrum—they live side by side, often in the same twelve-hour shift. And somewhere in that tension, we keep showing up.

Let me take you through two hours of night shift—0500–0700.

The tail end of the night shift, known to us as *the witching hour*. And no, I'm not talking about the witching hour of newborns. Every seasoned night nurse knows *this* is when the chaos peaks. Without fail, the most critical, high-stakes cases flood into the ER—devastating MVA's, cardiac arrests, overdoses. And it always hits at this hour. I don't know why. Maybe it's when people wake up and find their loved ones unresponsive? Maybe it's just bad luck? But by now, I've come to expect it and brace myself for what's to come.

That night, we had five intubations within a thirty-minute span: three cardiac arrests, one drug overdose, and one drug withdrawal.

Back to back to back to back to back.

While overdoses undoubtedly pose immediate, life-threatening risks, drug withdrawal can often be far more insidious and terrifying. Abruptly discontinuing substance use—known as going "cold turkey"—without a tapering plan or medical supervision, can lead to profound physical and psychological distress. This is especially true with substances like alcohol, benzodiazepines, and opioids. The rapid onset of withdrawal can bring about a cascade of severe symptoms, including seizures, cardiac complications, delirium, and in the most extreme cases, death. Alcohol and benzodiazepine withdrawal, for example, can trigger life-threatening conditions such as delirium tremens (DTs) or status epilepticus, both of which require urgent medical intervention. Unlike an overdose, where the danger is often more immediate, withdrawal symptoms can be subtle at first, frequently misattributed to other medical conditions. As time passes, however, these patients can deteriorate quickly, requiring interventions like intubation. Gradual tapering under medical supervision is *vital,* as it not only alleviates withdrawal symptoms but also significantly reduces the risk of catastrophic complications.

And if that wasn't enough, we were critically understaffed—both in personnel and resources.

One phlebotomist. One lab tech. One respiratory therapist—for the entire hospital. Four nurses to manage a thirty-two-bed emergency department. Within minutes, five ventilators were in use—patients sedated, tubes secured. The unit pulsed with purposeful motion. There was no time to process the gravity of what was unfolding—not yet. While much of the world was just beginning to stir, sipping coffee and preparing for the morning commute, we were deep in the trenches, navigating the fragile threshold between life and death—five times over.

"It's usually not this bad. We're just short-staffed tonight. I promise—it gets better."

You hear it often, usually said to the newest nurse, like a line passed down through generations of burned-out staff trying to offer hope. But over time, the words start to ring hollow—more a coping phrase than a comforting truth. A quiet anthem of a system stretched too thin.

As the night folds in on itself, hour after hour, the chaos becomes routine. And somewhere in the haze of alarms and adrenaline, the job starts to chip away at you. You begin to wonder if the passion that brought you here can withstand the weight of what it's become.

We stabilized the first patient—a cardiac arrest of an elderly male found unresponsive by his daughter at home. CPR initiated, code medications given, ROSC achieved, intubate. Then rolled right into the next room and did it again. And again. Then EMS brought in the withdrawal, and we repeated the process again.

Every alarm blaring. Every resource tapped. Every set of hands spoken for.

Five intubated patients—by the standard protocol, that should have meant five nurses. But remember, we only had four, and twenty-seven other beds still required care. In that moment, "standard of care" was a luxury we couldn't afford.

You keep your head down. You move quickly. You compartmentalize. You triage your compassion and your time. *How much of myself can I give to each of my patients?* And yes, the lower-acuity patients get frustrated—rightfully so. They scream your name in the halls, ask when you're coming back and why it's been so long. And all you can do is apologize and try to keep going.

Because there's no other choice.

Yet for all the overwhelming moments that threaten to drain you, there are those rare instances that spark a light— when you witness a life saved, a moment of clarity, or a glimmer of newfound self-confidence that reminds you why you push forward.

There's no guarantee we'll ever see a patient's recovery in real time. In fact, it's something we rarely get to witness. As frontline workers, we're trained to assess, stabilize, and make decisions that can tip the scales between life and death. I call it "the immediate"—where our minds take root. Once our work is done, we pass the baton and move on to "the next immediate," often never knowing what happens after we've done our part. But sometimes—just sometimes—we do.

A forty-two-year-old woman was wheeled into the ER, her face a portrait of fear. She had developed right-sided weakness, numbness, facial drooping, and slurred speech approximately one hour prior to arrival. EMS had received the call from her husband, who found her sitting on the couch, struggling to speak and in a daze. In a panic, he immediately called 911, unsure of what was happening but knowing something was terribly wrong.

"What brings you in today?" I asked, leaning in to reassure her. Though I already knew the answer, this question was as much about assessing her level of orientation as it was about gathering any additional subjective data.

Her eyes locked onto mine, a silent plea for comfort. But her only response was a single, desperate word: "No."

"How old are you?"

Again, the blank stare. Then, the soft whisper, "No."

In neurologic assessments, it is essential to differentiate between the two primary types of aphasia: Broca's aphasia and Wernicke's aphasia. Broca's aphasia, as demonstrated by this patient, is characterized by impaired language *production*. While individuals with Broca's aphasia typically retain the ability to understand both spoken and written language, their capacity to form words and construct coherent sentences is significantly impaired. In other words, they can understand you clearly but struggle to find the words to respond. In contrast, Wernicke's aphasia allows individuals to speak fluently, yet their speech often lacks meaning or coherence, accompanied by significant difficulties in *comprehension*. Essentially, they can speak, but it's meaningless.

Given her presentation and our clinical assessment, it was immediately apparent she was likely experiencing a stroke. A Code Stroke was called without hesitation. But as protocol demands, we couldn't rely on presumptions alone—we had to rule out conditions that can closely mimic cerebrovascular events.

In our minds, the neurologic and endocrine file cabinets flew open—each drawer offering a cascade of questions to ask and assessments to perform. Head trauma. Drug toxicity.

Hypoglycemia. Each possibility was reviewed and ruled out in rapid succession. The team moved with practiced urgency, making the processes of exclusion and confirmation unfold almost in parallel.

A CT scan confirmed an ischemic stroke, and with all criteria met, tissue plasminogen activator (tPA)—a potent fibrinolytic—was administered within the hour.

> In the treatment of acute ischemic stroke, hospitals commonly rely on alteplase, a potent fibrinolytic agent, to dissolve existing clots in patients who present within 4.5 hours of symptom onset— provided they meet specific criteria. When administered intravenously, alteplase is rapidly absorbed into the systemic circulation, where it acts through a dual mechanism at both the cellular and systemic levels. Its short half-life of approximately three to five minutes highlights the need for continuous infusion or repeated bolus dosing to maintain therapeutic plasma concentrations. Pharmacodynamically, alteplase works by selectively binding to fibrin within thrombi, catalyzing the conversion of plasminogen to plasmin, and facilitating fibrinolysis and clot destruction.

One of the most remarkable aspects of administering tPA is that, on rare occasions, you can witness its effects unfold almost immediately. It's as though a dimmed light is slowly being rekindled. Her speech began to form again—first fragmented, then full sentences. Her expressions grew clearer. Awareness returned to her gaze. It was a profound transformation, equally clinical and deeply personal in its significance. And as I watched it unfold, I felt something rare in the fast pace of emergency medicine—an overwhelming sense of awe.

She was later admitted for observation, as protocol requires. But for once, we were given the rare privilege of witnessing the moment when intervention becomes resolution—leaving you with the realization, *Damn, I was part of that.*

You can watch a person regain their speech, feel the pulse return while a family pleads for us to save them, or catch an incredibly rare disease before the doctor even notices—each moment brings its own kind of joy. Of satisfaction. Sure, those are the feel-good moments that remind you why you keep choosing this career. The visual proof of our work, showcased for the world to see. It's *tangible* joy, the kind you can point to and say, *I helped make that possible.* But there's another kind of joy in nursing—pure and raw—that funnels deep into my soul. It's not seen from the outside but rather a private, internal reminder of why I chose this career in the first place.

This kind of joy comes when you have the opportunity to see nursing again through fresh eyes—eyes that haven't yet been clouded by the weight of years in the field. It's like watching someone breathe fresh air for the first time. They approach each case with a curiosity that reignites my own. The questions they ask, the eagerness to learn, the wonder at the complexity of human physiology—it brings me back to the roots of my own journey, when I first chose this career with the same wide-eyed enthusiasm.

In those moments, I remember what it feels like to *love* nursing—not just as a job but as a passion. The field can often become robotic, and it's not our fault. It's the system, the pressures, the demands, and the way we are sometimes treated that can leave us feeling numb to the job. But when I see a student's eyes light up with understanding or pride after mastering a simple skill or connecting the dots, I realize that, in teaching them, I'm also teaching myself—how to love nursing again, how to celebrate the little wins, how to stay curious and agile.

And perhaps that's the ultimate paradox of nursing: The more we give, the more it takes. The deeper we dive into the lives of others, the more we become aware of our own vulnerabilities, our own limits. Burnout creeps in—not because we lack resilience, but because we've given all we can and then some. We come face-to-face with our humanity—both as caregivers and as individuals who, in the end, are just as fragile as the patients we care for.

But here's the thing: Joy and burnout are not opposing forces. They are intertwined, coexisting in a way that is uncomfortable, yes, but profoundly real. The burnout, with its weight and weariness, forces us to acknowledge our limits— to recognize that we are not invincible, that we cannot save everyone. It humbles us. It teaches us to give with awareness, to pace ourselves, to learn to set boundaries, even when everyone around us begs for more.

But in that same breath, joy slips in, quietly, unexpectedly. It comes not as an antidote to burnout but as a companion to it. It's in the smile of a patient you've fought so hard to stabilize. It's in the deep, appreciative nod of a colleague who sees your effort and shares your struggle. It's in the fleeting, sacred moments of connection that remind us why we endure. Without burnout, those moments of joy wouldn't carry the same weight. Instead, we would have celebrated the joys without understanding what it took to earn them.

In a way, burnout reminds us of our humanity, and joy reminds us of our purpose. We can't have one without the other. So we keep showing up. Not because it's easy, not because it's perfect, but because in the space between burnout and joy, we find reason. And that, in the end, is enough.

Conclusion

When I first began writing this book, I wasn't sure if anyone would want to read the messier parts of a nursing journey—the moments we tend to tuck away or try to forget. But I also knew those were the exact stories that needed to be told. To put down on paper. To discuss. To navigate the thoughts behind them. To debrief. This book was never about showcasing perfection. It was about pulling back the curtain and saying, *This is what it really feels like. This is what I've carried.*

At its core, *Debrief* is a reflection. A pause. A place to breathe and acknowledge that behind every badge is a human being—with emotions, doubts, successes, and regrets. The purpose of this book has always been to normalize the complexity of this profession, to give language to the things we often leave unsaid, and to create space for connection through shared experience.

Throughout these pages, I've revisited the defining moments that shaped the nurse—and person—I've become. I've reopened wounds I once tried to bandage too quickly, without the care of a proper debrief. From the weight of grief to the sting of betrayal to the quiet victory of finding my voice, each story was written with intention: to honor the lesson it carried, the emotion it stirred, or the shift it created in me. Together, they paint a portrait of a profession that is as deeply human as it is heroic. While each chapter stands alone, they all circle back to the same invitation: to pause, reflect, and learn.

This book wasn't written to give you answers. It was written to invite you into conversation—with yourself, with your colleagues, and with this calling we share. Because if we're going to keep showing up in this field, we owe it to ourselves to make space for the kind of growth that only comes when we stop, take a breath, and truly debrief.

If you remember anything from this book, let it be this: Your humanity is not a weakness—it's your greatest strength. The ability to feel deeply, to question, to struggle, and *still* return to the work with compassion is what makes you a *remarkable* nurse.

To the new graduates or those about to take that leap into practice: Give yourself grace to grow into the feeling of competence. The path to confidence isn't a straight line—it's filled with challenges, mistakes, and moments of doubt (as you've clearly seen throughout this entire book). But with each experience, you are becoming. Remember that.

To the veteran nurses: Never underestimate the power you hold—in the aura you exude, in the way you communicate, and in the words you choose. *You* shape the next generation. New nurses are watching you, learning from you, and looking up to you, whether you realize it or not. Remember what it felt like to walk in those first, uncertain steps and the role others played in your growth. Your kindness, patience, and guidance can make all the difference.

And for everyone: You don't have to carry it all alone. You don't need to have it all figured out. But you do owe it to yourself to pause, process, and honor your own experience. That's where real growth lives—in the debrief.

If you want to follow my journey, share a little of your own, or simply need a safe space with people who get it, you can find it here:

On social at **@stephaneebeggs**,

or at **RNExplained.com**.

About the Author

Stephanee Beggs, MSN-Ed, RN, is a registered nurse, educator, and entrepreneur whose candid insights into the nursing profession have resonated with millions. While preparing for the national licensure exam (NCLEX) at the height of the COVID-19 pandemic, she shared a spontaneous teaching video that quickly went viral—giving rise to RNExplained, her now multimillion-dollar educational platform.

Launched in June 2020—the same year she graduated from nursing school—RNExplained began as a humble side hustle, with Beggs hand-lettering nursing study sheets using ink pens and Crayola markers. Those early sheets laid the foundation for what is now a fully developed nursing education brand offering her bestseller, *The Nursing School Comprehensive Bundle*—a more than three-hundred-page spiral-bound guide covering eight core nursing classes, alongside pharmacology flashcards inspired by her experience teaching as adjunct faculty, badge reference cards, merchandise, and a fully accredited IV skills certification course offering two CE credits.

Since its launch, RNExplained has grown into a trusted global resource for nursing students and professionals alike.

But Beggs's mission has always gone beyond merely selling resources—she's deeply committed to authenticity and connection. What began as anonymous hands teaching on camera eventually evolved into full-face videos, personal storytelling, and professional wisdom drawn from her time on the frontlines of healthcare. Her content blends evidence-based teaching with real-world experience, delivered in a tone that's both relatable and rooted in clinical credibility. Beggs believes students don't just deserve quality content—they deserve to know the person *behind* the content.

In 2023, Beggs earned a coveted spot on the *Forbes* 30 Under 30 list in Education—recognition that validated her mission to make nursing education more accessible, relatable, and effective for learners worldwide. As the first registered nurse ever honored in the Education category, she was celebrated for her innovative teaching methods and use of digital platforms to close gaps in traditional nursing education.

Beggs's influence extends beyond the nursing community and into national media and high-profile health events. She has appeared on *Fox News* and *Business Insider* in on-camera interviews discussing the growth of her business and offering firsthand insight into the realities of nursing amid nationwide strikes. In 2025, she walked the red carpet at the American Heart Association's Red Dress Collection Concert, supporting the campaign to raise awareness of cardiovascular disease— the leading cause of death among women. That same year, she attended the Time100 Impact Dinner as a guest of FIGS, joining an evening dedicated to honoring the world's most influential health leaders and advancing global conversations around innovation in healthcare.

At her core, Beggs loves directly interacting with students, which led her to teach pharmacology to sophomore nursing students in the traditional BSN program at her alma mater, Mount Saint Mary's University. She drew on her own struggles with pharmacology to develop a teaching approach focused on clarity and connection. Rather than overwhelming students with isolated facts, Beggs's philosophy prioritizes understanding the "what" and "why" behind each medication and patient condition. Being face to face with learners deepened her skills as an educator and mentor, while also exposing gaps in nursing education that fuel her ongoing advocacy.

When she's not immersed in medicine, Beggs embraces an active outdoor lifestyle—though she admits hiking and camping aren't her favorites. You're more likely to find her by the beach or pool, taking "hot girl walks," or practicing Pilates. Sundays are dedicated to a cherished routine of visiting local farmers markets to select fresh produce, followed by baking inspired by her mother's culinary influence. Cooking and baking together were core to her childhood, filled with weekly recipe tastings and celebrations that brought family and friends together—like the twenty-first-birthday cakes her mom lovingly baked for all her best friends.

Beggs's background includes some unexpected chapters: She spent much of her childhood in Las Vegas, where her mother was a professional blackjack player. Among her fondest memories are playing *Pretty Pretty Princess* with her grandparents and wakeboarding at Lake Mead. She once played guitar, has broken fifteen bones (yes, she was a clumsy kid), and has a strong interest in learning piano and obtaining her Pilates certification—because, as she jokes, what else can she throw on her plate? She earned a bachelor's degree in business marketing and worked in corporate America before deciding to pursue nursing—little did she know, that choice would intertwine her passion for healthcare with her entrepreneurial spirit. Sharing these personal stories with her online audience helps Beggs connect authentically with her community.

As Beggs continues to grow RNExplained and expand her impact on nursing education, she remains deeply committed to fostering a supportive, transparent community for nurses and students alike. She continues to redefine what it means to be a nurse, empowering viewers to embrace their unique journeys and find the lesson in every trial and triumph. Her platform isn't just a resource—it's a movement to make nursing feel less intimidating and more human (with a dash of her wonderfully chaotic life along the way).

Follow Stephanee:
Instagram: @stephaneebeggs
TikTok: @stephbegg
Website: RNExplained.com
YouTube: @rnexplained